PHLEBOTOMY

FROM Student TO Professional

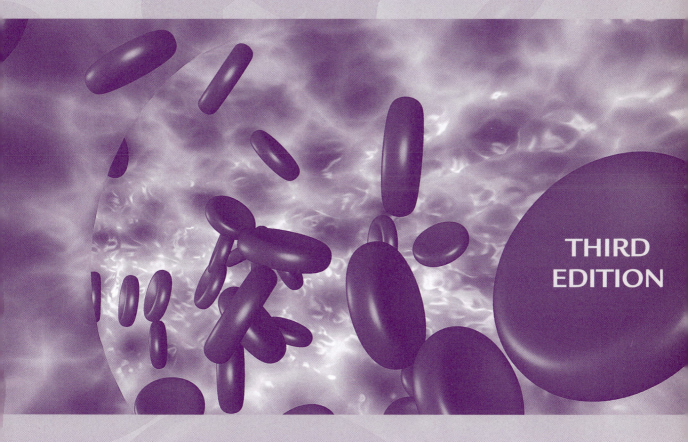

THIRD EDITION

BONNIE K. DAVIS

PHLEBOTOMY

FROM Student TO Professional

THIRD EDITION

BONNIE K. DAVIS

M.A. in Education, CLP (NCA), RPT (AMT)

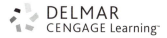

DELMAR
CENGAGE Learning™

Australia • Brazil • Japan • Korea • Mexico • Singapore • Spain • United Kingdom • United States

DELMAR
CENGAGE Learning™

Phlebotomy: From Student to Professional, Third Edition
Bonnie K. Davis, M.A., CLP (NCA), RPT (AMT)

Vice President, Career and Professional Editorial: Dave Garza

Director of Learning Solutions: Matthew Kane

Senior Acquisitions Editor: Sherry Dickinson

Managing Editor: Marah Bellegarde

Product Manager: Laura J. Wood

Editorial Assistant: Anthony R. Souza

Vice President, Career and Professional Marketing: Jennifer Ann Baker

Marketing Director: Wendy E. Mapstone

Senior Marketing Manager: Nancy Bradshaw

Marketing Coordinator: Erica Ropitzky

Production Director: Carolyn Miller

Content Project Manager: Allyson Bozeth

Senior Art Director: David Arsenault

For product information and technology assistance, contact us at
Cengage Learning Customer & Sales Support, 1-800-354-9706
For permission to use material from this text or product,
submit all requests online at **www.cengage.com/permissions**
Further permissions questions can be e-mailed to
permissionrequest@cengage.com

Library of Congress Control Number: 2010931649

ISBN-13: 978-1-4354-6957-0

ISBN-10: 1-4354-6957-7

Delmar
5 Maxwell Drive
Clifton Park, NY 12065-2919
USA

Cengage Learning is a leading provider of customized learning solutions with office locations around the globe, including Singapore, the United Kingdom, Australia, Mexico, Brazil, and Japan. Locate your local office at:
international.cengage.com/region

Cengage Learning products are represented in Canada by Nelson Education, Ltd.

To learn more about Delmar, visit **www.cengage.com/delmar**

Purchase any of our products at your local college store or at our preferred online store **www.cengagebrain.com**

Printed in the United States of America
1 2 3 4 5 6 7 12 11 10

Dedication

To my Family:
Ronnie, Rona, Ginny, Marty, Mom, and Dad with great love.

To my students and former employees with love and respect.

To my friends and colleagues:
Phyllis Austin, Susie Whitman, Jessica Nolting,
Vicki Bond, and Linda Tolan with gratitude and fond memories.

Contents

PART THREE

Professional Success in Phlebotomy / 185

CHAPTER 11

Communication Skills for the Phlebotomist / 186

CHAPTER 12

Conflict Management Skills / 196

CHAPTER 13

Becoming a Professional / 204

LIST OF PROCEDURES

Preface

Today's health care consumer demands and expects high-quality care. For the phlebotomist, that means having expert technical skills, a professional appearance and demeanor, and the ability to interact with customers in an effective, service-oriented manner. The quality of the phlebotomist's service creates a lasting impression on the customer-whether internal or external. Phlebotomy must be performed by well-trained professionals. This textbook is designed to prepare phlebotomy students in all aspects of blood sample collection, while emphasizing the importance of delivering this service in a customer-conscious manner. In addition, students are provided with information that will aid them in becoming employed. The textbook is designed with a community college curriculum as the standard. Emphasis is placed upon the student from success in the classroom to success as a professional.

PURPOSE OF THIS BOOK

I wrote this textbook with the purpose of providing prospective phlebotomists, laboratory technicians, nurses, and other health care workers with the necessary information and insight to become a successful professional in the area of laboratory specimen collection. The text is intended for formal classroom lectures combined with clinical laboratory applications. It is written in a concise, unpretentious language that gives students with no previous health care experience or previous health care education the opportunity to easily understand specimen collection procedures and techniques.

ORGANIZATION OF THIS BOOK

The book is divided into three parts. Part I introduces "Student Success in Phlebotomy." Chapter 1 describes the student's role in the classroom. The student is introduced to the phlebotomist's role in the health care environment, both past and present. This chapter is designed to give the phlebotomist a sense of identity that connects with the various disciplines in medicine. It will also help give the phlebotomist greater respect for and a sense of pride in the discipline of phlebotomy. Study tips, testing guidelines, and an overview of health care professionals and clinical laboratory departments give the student a strong basic foundation for success. Instructor expectations and clinical laboratory expectations are discussed. Chapter 2 covers the student's role in the clinical environment. Critical safety issues for the phlebotomist are examined in detail, including the role of OSHA, biological hazards, and chemical, electrical, and radiation safety. The student's role in customer service concludes the chapter.

Part II is on "Blood and Urine Collection." Chapter 3 discusses the circulatory system and serves as an important reference for the phlebotomist who is beginning to learn about blood collection. Chapter 4 covers blood collection equipment. Chapters 5 and 6 discuss collection by venipuncture and capillary puncture. Chapter 7 addresses special procedures such as blood cultures, glucose tolerance testing, and bleeding times. Chapter 8 covers special collection considerations such as newborn care, pediatric care, geriatric considerations, unsuccessful venipunctures, hand vein venipuncture, foot and ankle venipuncture, and point-of-care testing. Chapter 9 discusses the urinary system and laboratory testing of urine. Chapter 10 addresses common laboratory tests, including 50 blood and non-blood specimen requirements.

Part III focuses on "Professional Success in Phlebotomy." The phlebotomist is instructed in how to incorporate specimen collection techniques with customer service so that new skills are delivered in a customer-conscious manner. Chapter 11 discusses communication as it relates to phlebotomists. The phlebotomist's roles as a speaker and a listener are covered. An overview of appropriate telephone techniques is also provided. Chapter 12 discusses the daily conflicts that the phlebotomist encounters and provides instruction in how to analyze and solve conflicts. Chapter 13 is designed to help the student in becoming a professional. The transition from student to professional is emphasized, and there are guidelines for becoming a valuable and successful professional in today's challenging and competitive health care environment.

The learning aids that enhance the text can act as effective teaching tools as well. Chapter objectives are presented at the beginning of each chapter. They emphasize the important facts and topics to be covered and can be used as a framework to which additional material may be added as the chapter is read. Key terms are also presented at the beginning of each chapter. These are lists of some of the most important new words to be learned, and the terms appear in boldface type where they are explained in the text. Terms and definitions are also collected in the glossary in the back of the book for easy reference. Review activities are presented at the end of each chapter. The reviews cover the chapter content systematically and require students to answer in their own words by using "fill-in-the-blank" questions rather than multiple choice. An online resource provides answers to the review questions and a proficiency checklist.

NEW FEATURES IN THIS EDITION

The primary purpose of students who enroll in a phlebotomy course or phlebotomy certificate program is to obtain knowledge and technical skills necessary to become employed as a health care worker. Perhaps today's difficult economy has created a need for new job training. Or, perhaps there is a need for the students to bring in additional income into their household. Today's students may have limited funds and limited time to be trained and become employable. Upon completion of class courses, they hope to immediately to take their national certification examination, and be ready to start their job search. Because of these needs, this text has added tips and guidelines for becoming a successful student. Many students have not recently been in a formal classroom environment, and need help in becoming acclimated. The book also provides the student with tips and guidelines advice for job searches. In addition, there are guidelines in how to become a successful professional and maintain successful employment.

The most updated phlebotomy procedures, safety standards, and specimen collection requirements have been added. Students may successfully complete their national certification examination by studying this updated textbook.

Many health care facilities require phlebotomists to collect urine specimens. A chapter has been added to cover this topic.

A new full color art insert has been added to enhance student understanding of color coded tube tops and medical symbols, such as the biohazard symbol.

Online Resources

Online student and instructor resources have been made available. The online instructor guide includes:

- Answers to chapter review questions
- Final exam questions
- Log on to login.cengage.com to access these instructor resources.

The online student guide includes:

- Symbols and units of measure applicable to a phlebotomist's duties
- Examples of phlebotomist job descriptions
- Procedures for taking vital signs
- List of continuing education Web sites applicable to phlebotomy
- Log on to www.cengagebrain.com to access these additional student resources.

ABOUT THE AUTHOR

Bonnie K. Davis, Master of Arts in Education, CLP (NCA), RPT (AMT), is currently a professor in the Health Sciences Division at Pikes Peak Community College in Colorado Springs, Colorado. She designed and implemented the curriculum for the college Phlebotomy Certificate Program in 1997. In addition, she was the laboratory support manager of a large national health care organization for 26 years. Bonnie has spoken at numerous conferences on various phlebotomy and customer service topics. She may be contacted at Bonnie.Davis@ppcc.edu.

Reviewers

Mildred K. Fuller, Ph.D., MT (ASCP)
Allied Health Department
Chair and Professor
Norfolk State University
Norfolk, Virginia

James Hearn (Jay), CLS (NCA)
Health and Life Science
Phlebotomy Instructor
Athens Technical College
Athens, Georgia

Vyhyahn Maloof, MD
Medical and Public Services Department
Phlebotomy Program Director
Griffin Technical College
Griffin, Georgia

Joyce Stone, H(ASCP)SH
Contract Faculty
Lecturer
University of New Hampshire
Durham, New Hampshire

Judith Zappala
Adjunct Faculty
Middlesex Community College
Lowell, Massachusetts

Student Success in Phlebotomy

1

The Student's Role in the Classroom

OBJECTIVES

After studying this unit, it is the responsibility of the learner to be able to:

1. Explain the two primary roles of the phlebotomist.
2. Describe the five techniques used in bloodletting.
3. Discuss the history of phlebotomy.
4. Define professionalism.
5. Give examples of how personal qualities must be integrated into professional conduct.
6. Describe the professional appearance of the phlebotomist.
7. Define ethics.
8. Give examples of five ethical theories and how they affect the phlebotomist's role.
9. Define values.
10. List the components of The Patient Care Partnership issued by the American Hospital Association.
11. Discuss the difference between HIPAA and patient rights.
12. List five ways the phlebotomist may apply HIPAA to the patient's privacy.
13. Define patient confidentiality.
14. State the protocol for handling a patient's refusal to have a blood sample collected.
15. List the steps in completing an incident report.
16. List and describe the departments of the laboratory.
17. List tips for good study skills.
18. State the expectations of the clinical internship for phlebotomy students.

"*Whoever is to acquire a competent knowledge of medicine, ought to be possessed of the following advantages: a natural disposition; instruction; a favorable position for the study; early tuition; love of labour; leisure. First of all, a natural talent is required; for, when Nature opposes, everything else is vain; but when Nature leads the way to what is most excellent, instruction in the art takes place, which the student must try to appropriate to himself by reflection, becoming an early pupil in a place well adapted for instruction. He must also bring to the task a love of labour and perseverance, so that the instruction taking root may bring forth proper and abundant fruits.*"

—**Hippocrates**

antecubital before the crease of the forearm and upper arm

arterial puncture puncture of the radial, femoral, or brachial artery with the purpose of obtaining an arterial blood sample for testing pH, O_2, and CO_2

arteriotomy an incision into an artery

basilic vein blood vessel of the forearm that is acceptable for venipuncture

battery intentionally touching a person without authorization to do so

capillary puncture also called a skin puncture; this refers to puncturing the skin by means of a lancet to obtain a blood sample. This sample is a mixture of blood from arterioles, venules, and capillaries.

clot a clump of material formed out of the contents of blood

confidentiality the protected right of health professionals not to disclose information pertaining to a patient that is obtained during the delivery of health care services

cupping a technique of bloodletting where a vacuum is induced into a cup or glass. The glass is placed over the skin and the vacuum brings blood to the surface. The skin is cut and blood is allowed to flow.

cytopathology the science involved with disease at the cellular level

deontology an ethical theory based on moral obligation or commitment to others

egoism an ethical theory that considers self-interest the goal of all human actions

ethics an area of philosophy that examines values, actions, and choices to determine right and wrong

HIPAA Health Insurance Portability and Accountability Act; a federal protection law for the privacy of health insurance

histopathology science involved with the disease of tissue

humors fluids in the body

leech a blood-sucking worm utilized in bloodletting

ligate to tie a blood vessel with silk thread, wire, or filament to stop bleeding

morning rounds a batch of laboratory test orders scheduled for early morning collection

obligationism an ethical theory that attempts to resolve ethical dilemmas by balancing distributive justice with the promotion of good and the prevention of harm

phlebotomist an individual trained and skilled in obtaining blood samples for clinical testing

polycythenia abnormal increase in the number of erythrocytes in the blood

portal vein a short vein that receives branches from several veins leading from abdominal organs and then enters the liver

pulmonary circulation blood vessels transporting blood between the lungs and the heart

quality assurance established policies and procedures to ensure that laboratory testing is carefully monitored from beginning to end, including collection of specimens

risk management the monitoring of patterns and trends in the health care environment to assure the safety of patients and professionals

social contract theory an ethical theory based on the assumption that the least advantaged are the norm, with income, liberty, opportunity, and self-respect distributed equally

teleology an ethical theory that determines right or good based on an action's consequences

values strongly held personal and professional beliefs about worth and importance

venipuncture a puncture of a vein with the purpose of withdrawing blood

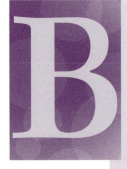ecoming a member of a health care team as a **phlebotomist** requires both technical skills and special personal qualities. *Webster's New International Dictionary of the English Language* defines phlebotomy as "the letting of blood in the treatment of disease." Even though the definition is overly concise, it does accurately describe the primary technical role of the phlebotomist. A phlebotomist obtains blood samples for laboratory testing by means of **venipuncture** (drawing blood from a vein), **arterial puncture** (drawing blood from an artery), and **capillary puncture** (obtaining blood from a capillary bed). Many hospitals do not require phlebotomists to perform arterial punctures. However, there are some special areas that may utilize the phlebotomist to obtain arterial specimens, such as emergency departments, outpatient labs, and the like. There are also some phlebotomy technician-certifying exams that require at least the knowledge of arterial punctures, such as the American Society of Clinical Pathologists (ASCP).

Phlebotomists may also work in situations that require collection of urine specimens and throat cultures. All collection procedures must be performed in such a manner as to ensure specimen integrity while causing minimal trauma to the patient. Patient and specimen identification must also be ensured by the phlebotomist throughout the collection process. The phlebotomist is responsible for collecting adequate volumes of blood in the appropriate collection tubes so as to provide the medical technologist who performs the testing with the best possible sample. These functions must be performed at a skill level that will provide quality service to both the laboratory and the patient.

In addition to technical skills, the phlebotomist must possess special personal qualities applicable to many professions in the business of providing service to a patient. In health care, there are several patients to which the phlebotomist will provide service: the patient, the patient's family and friends, the physician, coworkers, and other departments within the health care setting. The phlebotomist must be able to deliver technical skills to patients in such a manner as to promote goodwill and a desire in the patient to continue the service relationship.

A phlebotomist must be knowledgeable, compassionate, patient, friendly, a good listener, a good communicator, assertive, tolerant, honest, and energetic. Of course, these are all positive qualities that are desired for all service providers. However, for the phlebotomist, personal qualities must be combined with the sincere desire to work directly with people. A phlebotomist will spend each day working directly with patients and other members of the health care team. A person wishing to become a phlebotomist should ask himself or herself the following questions:

- Do I like people?
- Do I enjoy helping people?
- Can I take constructive criticism in a positive manner?
- Can I be polite when a patient is cross or rude?
- Can I be objective and calm in stressful moments?
- Am I willing to delay personal interests, such as rest breaks or going home on time, to meet patient needs?
- Am I willing to ensure quality patient care at all times? Am I willing to report errors in the best interest of the patient? Could I report errors even though they may have been made by myself or a friend?

If the answers to these questions are a resounding yes, and if you possess the personal qualities required for direct patient care, then you are a good candidate to begin a career as a phlebotomist.

■ PHLEBOTOMY IN THE PAST

Phlebotomy originated in ancient times, and was practiced in many cultures. It was a common practice in the treatment of disease until approximately 1860. At that time, phlebotomy for treatment of disease became an isolated practice. Over the past 60-plus years, phlebotomy has become a common procedure for collection of blood specimens for testing purposes.

To understand the history of phlebotomy, it is necessary to take a brief look at early medicine and the discovery of the circulatory system. Medicine has probably existed since the beginning of humanity. Primitive people believed that supernatural forces caused disease. Consequently, primitive medicine consisted of the practice of driving away the spirits that caused disease. Medicine was practiced and regulated by the Babylonians as early as 2250 B.C. Egypt was the birthplace of medical science. The Egyptians practiced medicine that was a combination of religion and superstition.

At the same time, they developed a very sophisticated form of medicine that would be used as a model for hundreds of years. The Egyptians performed surgical operations, prescribed various medicines, and performed religious healings. Egyptian medicine became the basis for Greek medicine.

Hippocrates (460–377 B.C.), who was known as the Father of Medicine, was the pupil of an Egyptian. Prior to the work of Hippocrates, Grecian medicine was in the hands of a religious organization, the priests of Asclepius. The priests believed that the gods brought disease, and only the gods could relieve it. Hippocrates separated medicine from religion. He developed a scientific medicine. Hippocrates supplied a philosophy and ethics that were the influences of future medicine. He introduced a rational approach to medicine by applying reasoning and objective observation. Hippocrates did not create the medical knowledge of his time. Instead, he took the knowledge and turned it into a science. He was the first to systematically record patient's symptoms and prepare clinical care histories. He then was able to define and classify diseases. Hippocrates established the procedure for diagnoses and prognoses.

Hippocratic doctrine developed the Humoral Theory, which said that disease was caused by an imbalance of the four bodily **humors**: blood, phlegm, yellow bile, and black bile. When blood is allowed to **clot** outside the body, four portions can be recognized in it: a dark clot, a red fluid, a yellow serum, and fibrin. Each of these was given a name related to a behavior pattern of the human being. The behavior pattern was believed to be caused by an excess of one of the portions of the blood clot, while health was a proper balance of the four humors. In addition, the four humors were subdivided into hot or cold, and dry or moist. By these elements a person's characteristics and personality were formed. The Humoral Theory of disease was held in one form or another by physicians until the middle of the nineteenth century.

Three hundred years after Hippocrates, Grecian medicine began to be practiced in Rome. Galen became the most notable physician of the Roman period. In fact, the period from Galen until the seventeenth century was dominated by Galenic medicine. The period from the seventeenth century onward has been dominated by the revival of Hippocratic medicine.

Galen (130–201 A.D.) became a renowned physician in Pergamum, and published writings on physiology and anatomy. Galen accepted an appointment as physician and surgeon to the gladiators. During his appointment, he was able to observe muscles, bones, and blood flow, which allowed him to develop the basis for his writings on surgical techniques. Galen discovered that inspired air entered the lungs during the act of breathing and was then mixed with the blood. But he believed that all the blood was formed in the liver and was brought from the intestines by the **portal vein**.

Blood was carried by way of the nerves, which he thought of as hollow tubes throughout the body. Previous to Galen's theory, Erasistratus had described the heart valves and traced the anatomy of the blood vessels. However, he concluded that the arteries in the body contained only air. Galen recognized that the arteries contained blood and not air. He recognized that the heart set the blood in motion, but he did not know that blood circulated. Galen believed that blood ebbed and flowed in the vessels.

It is amazing that Galen's concept of circulation was accepted without doubt until the Renaissance. At that time, Andreas Vesalius (1514–1564) revolutionized anatomy, and exposed the mistakes of Galen. Vesalius discovered the existence of **valves** in the veins, but did not understand their significance. Vesalius was followed by Realdus Columbus (1510–1599). Columbus discovered the **pulmonary circulation**. However, there was still no concept of circulation of the blood. A Spaniard, Michael Servetus (1509–1553), came close to discovering the circulation of blood. However, the ebb and flow idea still persisted.

William Harvey (1578–1657) is credited with the discovery of the circulatory system. Over 1600 years had passed since Galen proposed his concept of the circulatory system, and his ideas still were accepted as correct until Harvey's discoveries. William Harvey revolutionized medical science. He described the circulation of blood from observations on living animals and by dissections. Harvey demonstrated that the heart is a hollow muscle containing four chambers. He came to the conclusion after a long series of experiments in which he discovered that the pulse was due to the pounding of the heart rather than the throbbing of the veins. Harvey **ligated** the arteries and then divided them to prove that the arterial blood flowed away from the heart. Other experiments led him to discover that the auricles and ventricles on each side of the heart do not contract in unison, but instead, one contraction succeeds the other.

Harvey also discovered the function of the valves in the veins. He determined that the valves prevent a backflow of the blood toward the extremities, which keeps the blood in motion. Harvey was able to determine the function of the valves of the vein after studying the flow of blood in his own hand. One day as he was stroking the back of one hand with the finger of the other, he noticed that when stroking downward over the **basilic vein**, the blood was prevented from following the direction of his finger. However, when he released it, the blood immediately rushed up to fill the empty vein. Harvey decided that there must be a valve that prevented the blood from returning before the release.

The discovery of the circulatory system involved a long process. From Galen to Harvey, there were many beliefs and theories that proved false. Included in those errors was the use of bloodletting.

Bloodletting

A leading textbook of medicine written about 1840 said: "Of all the treatments in medicine, the most efficacious is the letting of blood: stand the patient upright and bleed from the **antecubital** vein until syncope occurs." Bloodletting was probably useful in some cases of hypertension and in **polycythenia**. However, it is likely that while it may not have always caused harm, it did not help in many cases and probably caused the death of many patients during the 3000 years that it was practiced. Regardless, it was an accepted and standard practice for releasing evil spirits, cleansing the body of impurities, adjusting excess body fluids, and treating a variety of diseases and ailments. Please see Figure 1-1 for the major bloodletting points utilized for bloodletting.

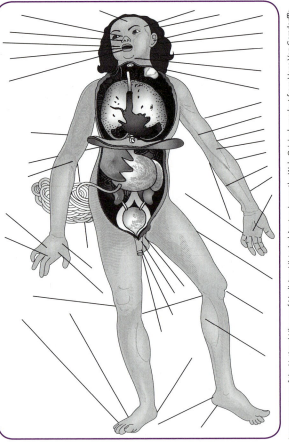

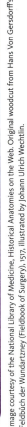

Image courtesy of the National Library of Medicine, Historical Anatomies on the Web. Original woodcut from Hans Von Gersdorff's Feldbúch der Wundartzney (Fieldbook of Surgery). 1517, illustrated by Johann Ulrich Wechtlin.

Figure 1-1 Bloodletting chart by Johann Ulrich Wechtlin, showing the positions of the major bloodletting points, based upon the teachings of Galen.

Bloodletting Instruments and Procedures

A variety of instruments were used over the centuries to perform bloodletting procedures. Early instruments included thorns, needles, sharp bones, sticks, flint, and shells. Miniature bow and arrow devices for bloodletting have been found in South America and New Guinea. A small bloodletting instrument resembling a crossbow was once used in Greece and Malta. Wall paintings dating from 1400 B.C. depict the use of leeches for drawing blood from human beings. As bloodletting practices advanced, a variety of instruments developed, which included lancets, scalpels, fleams, various cupping devices, and scarificators. Please refer to Figure 1-2a, Figure 1-2b, and Figure 1-2c.

The five techniques used for bloodletting are:

1. Venesection
2. Arteriotomy
3. Cupping
4. Scarification
5. Leeching

Venesection

Venesection was the most commonly used method for bloodletting. Lancets, scalpels, venesection knives, ink erasers, and fleams were the instruments used to perform venesection. Lancets had tortoise shell, ivory, or pearl folding guards. The cases were made of silver or tortoise shell, and resembled a pocket cigarette lighter in size and shape.

Spring lancets and spring fleams were introduced in 1680. They consisted of a single blade that was spring-loaded. The spring was encased within the body of the instrument. It was often made of brass and was

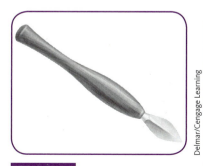

Figure 1-2a Scalpel Lancet

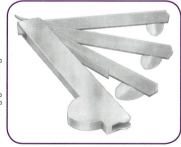

Figure 1-2b Many-bladed Fleam

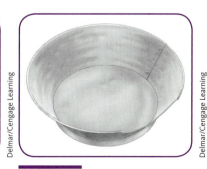

Figure 1-2c Bleeding Bowl

Delmar/Cengage Learning

5–8 cm in length. The point of the blade was withdrawn into the body of the instrument, the trigger or release lever was pressed, and the blade was released. The blade penetrated the skin and the vein.

The spring lancets were difficult to control. The incision was often too small or too large, and there was often injury to the tendon or nerve. An accidentally severed artery was not uncommon. Thus, the manually controlled lancets were preferred over the spring devices. The fleam was a generic term for several bloodletting tools. Basically it was an instrument with several blades that folded into a case. Each blade was a different size and was attached to a shaft at a right angle. Scalpels, venesection knives, and ink erasers were also used. They had the same appearance even though they had varied functions, including in surgery procedures and venesections, and as instruments to remove ink from paper.

The procedure for manually performing a venesection was similar to that in today's venipuncture. There was a tourniquet placed above the elbow. However, the lancet was inserted into the vein, and a small incision was made in an oblique manner, producing a cut the same length as the width of the vein. The blood was allowed to flow into a bowl for measurement.

For hundreds of years a circular household bowl was used to catch the blood. The bowls were used for a variety of purposes such as washing or shaving and were often made of metals such as copper, brass, tin, and pewter. It was difficult to measure the blood accurately with a large bowl, so often a small bowl was placed inside the larger bowl. About 1500 A.D. a circular notch was cut into the circumference of the bowl. This was done so that the notch could fit against the neck of the antecubital fossa. Bowls were also made of glass, skin, papier mâché, and wood. Some bowls were elaborately decorated. After the proper amount of blood was withdrawn, the tape tourniquet was removed, dry lint applied to the wound, and a bandage applied to hold the lint in place.

Arteriotomy

Arteriotomy was a less frequently used procedure for bloodletting. It was potentially a very dangerous method. It was usually performed on the superficial temporal artery or one of its branches. The artery was partially cut through a single incision. When the appropriate amount of blood was withdrawn, the artery was completely severed. The artery contracted and stopped the flow of blood. As with the venesection, dry lint was applied to the wound and a tight bandage placed over the lint.

Cupping

Dry and wet **cupping** involved a procedure that required placing a suction cup over an area of skin. Suction was applied to create a blister or swollen area. In the case of dry cupping, the blister or swollen area drew the underlying blood away from the inflamed area and directed it to the surface of the skin. The blood or fluid in the blister was not removed. Wet cupping involved cutting the skin so that blood and fluid could be extracted.

Scarification

Scarificators contained from 1 to 20 blades, and were similar in appearance to the lancet. Cupping devices were made of glass, a gourd, or an animal's horn. In the case of the horn, a small hole was made in the pointed end. The bloodletter placed the large opening of the horn on the patient's skin and sucked on the small opening to create suction. The mouth side was then covered with wax or an eggshell skin. Another method used to create suction involved heating the inside of the cupping glass. A burning torch was used to briefly heat the glass before it was placed on the patient's skin. Wet cupping is described in an 1860 textbook, *Modern Surgery*. The description of the equipment used includes a scarificator, cupping glass, torch, wine, candle, hot water, and sponge. The patient's skin was to be prepped by sponging with warm water and then dried. A torch soaked in wine was set on fire and used to heat the inside of the cupping glass for one second. The glass was immediately applied to the patient's skin and left until a red swollen area appeared. The glass was then removed and a scarificator used on the swollen area to perforate the skin. The cupping glass was reheated and placed over the perforated skin. Three to five ounces of blood was bled, and the wound was dressed with lint.

Leeching

Leeches were commonly used as early as 200 B.C. for bloodletting purposes. They were applied to the patient's skin on the affected area and allowed to fill themselves with blood. Leeches usually fell off when they became full of blood. If a larger amount of blood was to be let, the tail of the leech was simply cut off and the blood allowed to flow until the desired amount of blood was released.

The five different bloodletting methods—venesection, arteriotomy, cupping, scarification, and leeches—were used over a period of 3000 years throughout many cultures. The Chinese practiced bloodletting for many centuries. The instruments used were needles rather than knives. Needles ranged in size from a thin wire to a small scalpel.

Bloodletting is discussed frequently in medieval Jewish writings. It was used as a remedy for illness, but was used most frequently as a type of preventive medicine. Generally, the Talmudic view was that venesection was harmful if excessive, but useful if performed in an appropriate manner. The Talmud describes the instruments for bloodletting. A lancet, actually a small knife, was used to cut the skin. In addition, another pointed instrument that looked like a nail was used. The blood was allowed to flow on the ground or it was collected in a vessel called a Kadden, a potsherd, or a dirty earthenware vessel that was no longer unusable for its original purpose. Cupping glasses, made of both glass and horns, were also used by Talmudic sages.

Bloodletting was practiced by the Egyptians as early as 1000 B.C., and spread from there to the Greeks and Romans. Galen promoted the use of bloodletting in 200 A.D. It became a popular procedure practiced throughout the world. In Europe priests and monks became the primary practitioners of bloodletting, and retained that practice for over 1000 years. In 1163 A.D. a church edict prevented clergy from practicing bloodletting. At that time the barber-surgeon became the responsible party for bloodletting, dentistry, amputation of arms and legs, lancing of abscesses, and keeping of public baths, as well as hair cutting. They also performed coroner duties. The monks formed an alliance with the barbers shortly before 1100 A.D. The monks primarily supervised the barbers, who were the surgeons for the common people. It was during this time that the traditional barber pole originated. The pole actually had nothing to do with barbering, but instead is symbolic of surgery. The pole originated from the staff of authority carried by the physician from ancient times. The barber-surgeon carried the staff with a bandage attached to it, which was used for tying the patient's arm. Red and white stripes were painted on the staff with red symbolizing the let blood and white symbolizing the bandages. The barber-surgeon alliance continued until 1744. At that time, the barbers returned to hair cutting and the surgeons moved on to a more respected place in medicine.

During the thirteenth century, the use of bloodletting as a therapeutic treatment became increasingly popular. Bloodletting was used as a type of preventive medicine for healthy adults. The Talmud stated that venesection was to be included among the costs that a husband is obligated to pay for the continuing necessary medical treatment of his wife.

By the end of the 1700s, bloodletting was used very frequently with two purposes in mind: to reduce inflammation fever and to improve the quality of blood. It has been recorded that as much as 3600 cc of blood was withdrawn from a vein over a period of 7 hours. There was also a belief that there was an advantage in letting blood near the patient's head. Therefore, the jugular vein was often opened. Some practitioners believed that 900–1800 cc of blood was an adequate amount to withdraw if cups were applied to the temples and nape of the neck and, along with leeches, applied to the shaven scalp.

Bleeders continued to recklessly practice frequent and heavy bloodletting practices into the early nineteenth century. Benjamin Rush, a well-known eighteenth-century physician, maintained that bleeding should be repeated until symptoms disappeared, even if as much as four-fifths of the blood in the body was withdrawn. An example of reckless use of bleeding caused the death of George Washington. Washington died in 1799 as a result of voluminous bleeding. He was bled four times as a treatment for an upper respiratory tract infection. Estimates of the amount of blood lost by Washington as a result of bloodletting range from 5 to 9 pints.

The practice of bloodletting began to decline in the latter part of the nineteenth century. By 1860 it had basically disappeared from use in most hospitals. Today bloodletting is practiced primarily as a means for obtaining a blood sample to be used for diagnostic testing. However, blood removal for treatment may still be used in cases of polycythemia and hemochromatosis. Phlebotomy instruments have certainly changed throughout the years, but is amazing how similar the principle of collection remains.

The most used system for blood collection today is the evacuated blood collection system. The vacuum tube was first manufactured in the early 1920s by Hynson, Wescott, and Dunning. The system consisted of a sealed ampule connected to a rubber tube with a needle at the end. The phlebotomist performed the venipuncture, and then crushed the stem of the ampule. The vacuum in the ampule caused the blood to flow into the tube.

Bloodletting continues to be part of our medical practice. Its purpose and procedures have changed somewhat, but it endures. The history of the profession reveals that many things have not changed over thousands of years.

PROFESSIONALISM

Having the right personal qualities and a desire to serve are very important aspects in becoming a phlebotomist. However, they must be integrated into a standard of performance called professionalism. Professionalism is difficult to define. *Webster's New International Dictionary of the English Language* has several definitions listed under "profession" and "professionalism." The definition that will be used for this book is "conduct that manifests fine artistry or workmanship based on sound knowledge and conscientiousness."

The key word is *conduct*. The conduct of the phlebotomist is extremely important in providing quality patient care. The phlebotomist must remember that it is desirable to integrate those very important personal qualities of friendliness, compassion, and honesty with the standards of conduct required of a medical professional. For example, friendliness is very important when interacting with a patient, but if friendliness is not tempered with professionalism, there is a risk that the phlebotomist will become too friendly. Friendliness may take the form of invasion of privacy, because the phlebotomist asks inappropriate personal questions. Or friendliness may develop into a personal, intimate relationship that interferes with the delivery of patient care. In such a situation, the patient may feel free to ask the phlebotomist for test results that have not been reviewed by the physician. An intimate, personal relationship may lead the phlebotomist to make poor decisions. Giving a patient test results without a physician's authorization is not appropriate behavior.

The phlebotomist must maintain a balance between friendliness and sound medical service. A rule of thumb would be to do only what is in the patient's best interest. While the patient may want to be given test results, complying with this request may not be in the patient's best interest. Giving test results to a patient without the knowledge of the physician can have serious consequences. The patient may not be able to interpret the results or may have a very emotional response to results bearing bad news. A phlebotomist must always remember that his or her employer is liable for all professional actions. Other examples of integrating personal qualities with professional conduct follow.

Helpfulness

The phlebotomist should be helpful to the patient. However, medical advice is never to be given by the phlebotomist. The phlebotomist is not trained to "play doctor." In addition, a phlebotomist is never to tell a patient why a physician has ordered a particular test. The phlebotomist should give the patient the name of the test and refer the patient to the physician for further explanation.

Compassion

Empathy is a desired quality for a phlebotomist. It gives one an understanding of the fears and actions of the patient. A patient may fear needles because of a previous bad experience when having blood collected, and a particularly compassionate and skillful phlebotomist may then become the patient's favorite phlebotomist. However, the phlebotomist should not encourage a dependent relationship with the patient, for if the patient requires a blood sample to be drawn when the phlebotomist is not available, there will be problems for both the patient and the phlebotomist's coworkers.

Efficiency

It is very important to perform duties in such a manner as to ensure prompt and timely collections. Still, the phlebotomist must not rush through the collection process to the point that the patient is treated as an object. Holding a friendly conversation with the patient, in a pleasant tone of voice, is required no matter how quickly the sample must be collected. In addition, haste should never replace accuracy and quality. Careful attention to identifying the patient, labeling the specimen, and collecting the correct type of specimen and volume of blood must always be ensured.

Personal Appearance

In addition to conduct, another component of professionalism is personal appearance. While the behavior of the phlebotomist is a major part of the professional image, personal appearance also contributes to that image. A clean, well-groomed appearance is imperative for the phlebotomist. Although each health care facility has its own dress requirements, the following considerations should be included:

- Attire should be clean, fresh, and wrinkle-free. If white uniforms are required, the color should be a true white. Age tends to discolor white uniforms, making them appear dingy. New lab coats and uniforms should be purchased as soon as old ones take on this dinginess. Uniforms should also be in good repair. Clothing should fit comfortably and be the appropriate size.
- Shoes should be polished and in good condition.
- Hairstyles should be moderate.
- Personal hygiene is of utmost importance, because of the close proximity in which the phlebotomist works with the patient.
- Hands are the tools of the phlebotomist and are closely observed by patients. Nails should be clean and well manicured. Chipped nail polish should be removed immediately.
- Jewelry, cologne, perfume, and makeup should be worn in moderation. Some health care facilities ask phlebotomists not to wear fragrances, owing to patient allergies.

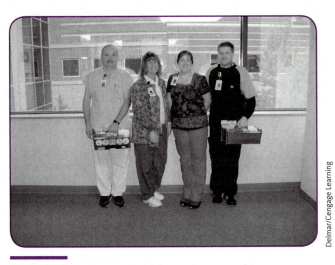

Delmar/Cengage Learning

Figure 1-3 Professional phlebotomy team.

Appearance makes an immediate impression on the patient and will determine the patient's confidence in the phlebotomist. Professional appearance and behavior will help the phlebotomist in performing the collection of the blood sample. Patients are much more cooperative when they have confidence in the phlebotomist Please refer to Figure 1-3 for a view of phlebotomists who maintain professional appearance.

■ ETHICS

It is important for the phlebotomist to maintain high professional standards. To do so requires some understanding of the ethics of the medical profession.

Ethics is the area of philosophical study that examines values, actions, and choices to determine right and wrong. The word *ethics* is derived from the Greek word *ethos,* which means a custom or practice, a distinguishing character or manner of acting. Since the beginning of time, when people have grouped together to satisfy a common need, they have set up rules. The strength and acceptance of these rules determine the strength and longevity of the society to which they pertain. The medical field is no different from any other society.

Ethics is composed of ethical theories. Ethical theories provide a system of principles and rules for resolving ethical dilemmas. In addition, the theories set forth fundamental beliefs about what is right and wrong, and suggest reasons for maintaining those beliefs. It is helpful for phlebotomists to know and understand basic ethical theories so that they may understand the foundation for the ethical requirements of their role as a phlebotomist. Because phlebotomists are members of a medical team, they must be aware of the rules by which the team functions.

The following are types of ethical theories:

1. **DEONTOLOGY** emphasizes moral obligation or commitment. An example of a moral commitment would be to always tell the truth. Deontology focuses on duty or obligation to others. An example specifically pertaining to the phlebotomist would be to admit to an error in identifying the patient if such an error has been made. The phlebotomist might suffer some consequences, but the patient's well-being would be more important. The phlebotomist would be expected to focus on the duty or obligation to the patient.

2. **TELEOLOGY** determines what is right or wrong based on an action's consequences. Ethical decisions are based on risk or benefit analysis. Another way of stating the theory would be to ask, "Does the good outweigh the bad?" An example relevant to the phlebotomist might concern the drawing of an emergency blood sample. If the phlebotomist tries twice to get the sample but does not succeed, would it be more beneficial for the phlebotomist to attempt additional venipunctures and deliver the specimen for testing in an expeditious manner? Or would it be more beneficial to ask for assistance from another phlebotomist, delaying the collection of the specimen? In this case, the phlebotomist would be making a benefit analysis of the situation.

3. **SOCIAL CONTRACT THEORY** is based on the concept that the least advantaged people in society (such as people with disabilities) are considered the norm. An act is determined right or wrong from the norm's point of view. For example, if there are two patients in the outpatient lab, and the first to arrive for routine lab tests is an indigent person while the second to arrive for routine lab tests is the spouse of the hospital CEO, which patient should receive priority treatment? The phlebotomist would be making a decision based on social contract theory if the first patient to arrive was taken care of first, regardless of other factors.

4. **EGOISM** considers self-interest and self-preservation to be the only goals behind all human actions. It does not consider moral principles outside the individual's point of view. It does not consider the rights of others. An example for the phlebotomist might be a case in which a newspaper offers to pay for confidential medical information concerning a nationally known political figure. The phlebotomist might choose to reveal the information

for monetary gain, even though the patient may be hurt by the action. This phlebotomist would be applying egoism theory.

5. **OBLIGATIONISM** balances the idea of "dividing equally" with that of "doing good and not harm." According to this theory, benefits and burdens should be distributed equally throughout society. People must be treated according to their merits and needs. An example for the phlebotomist would be the decision to collect emergency orders before routine ones.

An understanding of these basic ethical theories will help the phlebotomist visualize the big picture of professional standards in the medical field.

VALUES

It is important for phlebotomists to be aware of their own value systems, so they can understand feelings and actions when working within the medical environment. **Values** are strongly held personal and professional beliefs. The word *value* comes from the Latin *valere*, which means to be strong. Values may reflect positive or negative feelings. The following might be examples of phlebotomists' value statements:

· Phlebotomists are integral members of the health care team.
· Phlebotomists should be paid more for what they do.
· Phlebotomy is a skill.

Not all phlebotomists would agree with all of these value statements. Value conflicts are common among phlebotomists, as they are among other health care workers.

Understanding personal values is an important part of developing a professional ethic. Phlebotomists should clarify their own values and decide if they are consistent with ethical standards of the medical profession.

Finally, phlebotomists must know and understand the mission statement of their employer. Knowing the employer's mission statement and values helps to build teamwork, pride, and a sense of ownership among professionals.

PATIENT RIGHTS

An employer's mission statement will usually incorporate a statement of patients' rights. Phlebotomists need to know and understand patients' rights if they are to perform phlebotomy duties in an appropriate manner consistent with the medical profession. Today's phlebotomy patients are more knowledgeable and assertive than in the past, and they are more involved in decisions concerning their treatments. They are also more likely to initiate malpractice suits when the quality of care does not meet their expectations.

Phlebotomists must support their employer by knowing and ensuring appropriate, quality service. An understanding of patient rights and how they apply to the phlebotomist is important.

The American Hospital Association drafted a Patient's Bill of Rights in 1975. It listed 12 specifics rights of the patient when receiving care in the hospital. The bill was replaced in 2003 by the Patient Care Partnership. The Partnership was written to ensure greater satisfaction of the patient, physician, and health care facility by clarifying expectations, rights, and responsibilities of the patient and health care providers.

The patient may expect the following during their hospital stay:

- High quality hospital care
- A clean and safe environment
- Involvement of the patient in the patient's care
- Protection of privacy
- Help when leaving the hospital
- Help with billing claims

The hospital may expect from the patient:

- Accurate information about past hospitalizations, illnesses, medications, and other information concerning health matters
- Questions and requests for clarification when additional information is needed in order to participate in the healing process
- A copy of the patient's advance directive
- Reasonable requests regarding accommodations
- Necessary information for insurance claims and the provision of payment arrangements
- Recognition of the impact of lifestyle on personal health

Although the American Hospital Association has no enforcement mechanism, many hospitals use this statement as a model. If patients believe a hospital has violated their legal rights, they may take legal action. Whether a patient's rights statement is legally binding or not, the phlebotomist should consider patient's rights to be *professionally* binding. Phlebotomists must uphold and support the mission statements of their employer, governmental regulations, and professional organizations in the field.

HIPAA

Separate from the Patients' Bill of Rights, **HIPAA** provides for several patient rights. The Health Insurance Portability and Accountability Act of 1996 (HIPAA) is the first comprehensive federal protection law for the privacy of health information. It provides for patients' rights and control over their information by setting limits on the use and disclosure of their health information. In addition, it establishes safeguards to protect the privacy of the information in all forms, including paper records, oral communications, and electronic information. The final HIPAA Privacy Rule took place on April 14, 2003.

Before HIPAA, personal health information could be distributed to others without either notice or authorization from the patient. Because computers make information exchange so easy, laws had to be enacted to protect patient privacy. HIPAA provides for several patient rights, including these:

- The right to notice of a service provider's privacy practices
- The right to access health information
- The right to request restrictions on how health information is used and disclosed
- The right to request amendments or corrections to health information
- The right to accounting of disclosures

Phlebotomists should apply all patient rights to privacy by doing the following:

- Preserving, protecting, and safeguarding patient privacy and confidential health information at all times
- Not sharing patient information with others unless necessary for the treatment of the patient
- Not writing down computer passwords or sharing them with anyone
- Logging off the computer when leaving the work area so other students or professionals cannot use your password
- Using care when it is necessary or appropriate to discard patient health information. Confidential materials should be shredded.

Penalties for breaking the HIPAA privacy rules are twice the penalty for Medicare and Medicaid fraud and abuse. Breaching patient confidentiality and/or breaking the privacy policies and procedures will most likely lead to disciplinary action or perhaps even termination of your course of student clinical courses. Additionally, the federal government can impose monetary penalties as low as $100 per violation and up to $250,000 and 10 years in prison.

■ LEGAL ISSUES

Confidentiality

The main purpose of **confidentiality** is to encourage communication at an intimate level between a professional and a patient. According to *Principles of Biomedical Ethics,* "A rule of confidentiality prohibits (some) disclosures of (some) information gained in certain relationships to (some) third parties without the consent of the original source of information" (Beauchamp & Childress, 1989).

Confidentiality is important for professionals in many fields. Lawyers, teachers, counselors, and other professionals must be concerned with confidentiality. In a medical context, confidentiality in regard to a patient's diagnosis and prognosis is of utmost importance. Confidentiality excludes unauthorized persons from gaining access to patient information. In addition, it requires that people who do have access to privileged information refrain from communicating it to others. If patients do not believe that a physician or other health care professionals will maintain confidences, they may not supply personal information important for their care and treatment.

Frequently, many different health care workers need access to a patient's medical records in order to provide proper care. Phlebotomists will have access to such information as a patient's diagnosis, treatment plan, personal history, billing information, and so on. Such information is confidential. Even though the information is accessible, this does not mean that curiosity is a sufficient reason to open a patient's file. A phlebotomist must demonstrate self-discipline when dealing with patient information. The phlebotomist must be careful not to discuss confidential information in public areas such as cafeterias, halls, or elevators. Such conversations may be overheard by visitors, family members, and others. When patient cases are used as examples in classrooms or other teaching areas, care must be given to mask the identity of the patients. The phlebotomy student will be anxious to share daily activities with family and friends, but here, too, it is very important that the identity of patients not be disclosed. Confidentiality must be ensured to protect the patient.

[ALERT]

Patients have the right to refuse to have their blood drawn, even
if ordered by a physician. Comply with the patient's wish, and
do not collect a blood sample. Notify the appropriate nurse,
physician, or supervisor.

Refusal of Treatment

A patient may legally refuse treatment. A phlebotomist will experience
situations in which a patient refuses to have blood drawn. As a professional,
you must respect that decision. You should not argue with the patient
concerning this decision. Never ignore a patient's decision to refuse to
have blood collected and attempt to proceed regardless of that decision.
A patient can sue you for **battery**, which means intentionally touching
another person without authorization to do so. If a patient should refuse
to have blood drawn, you should follow these steps:

1. Explain to the patient that the doctor has ordered the tests and
   needs the test results for decisions regarding treatment.
2. If the patient continues to refuse, notify the physician and, if
   applicable, the patient's nurse.
3. Notify the appropriate person in your department.
4. Document the patient's refusal.

RISK MANAGEMENT AND QUALITY ASSURANCE

It is very important for phlebotomists to maintain high professional
standards of practice for themselves and for coworkers. Phlebotomists,
like all health care professionals, usually want to ensure accurate and
efficient work. Mistakes will happen, however. To address errors and
ensure top-quality care, hospitals have created mechanisms for monitoring
the quality of patient care. Such mechanisms fall under the categories of
risk management and **quality assurance**. Quality assurance may also be
referred to as continuous quality improvement, or CQI.

As a phlebotomist, you have a legal duty to report any inappropriate
incident of which you have direct knowledge. Specifically, a phlebotomist must be willing to take appropriate action to safeguard the patient if

incompetent or illegal actions are observed. Failure to report an incident may lead to termination of employment or even exposure to personal liability for malpractice.

Fear of negative peer pressure or of making the accused angry may make the phlebotomist apprehensive about reporting on a colleague. However, reporting inappropriate behavior can be carried out successfully if it is done in a systematic manner. The following process should be followed when reporting any illegal or incompetent behavior of a coworker:

1. Gather information. Complete an incident report.

2. Report the incident to the appropriate person, according to the employer's chain of command.

3. Maintain a record of efforts to report the incident through appropriate channels.

4. After a reasonable duration, determine whether the problem has been corrected.

5. If the problem still exists, report the incident to the person at the next level of command.

An incident report may be used to report other types of problems as well. An incident is an event that is inconsistent with ordinary procedure. For instance, any injury to a patient would require an incident report. Incident reports may also be used to document patient complaints, errors, and injuries to professionals and visitors. Phlebotomists have a legal duty to report any incident of which they have firsthand knowledge. Incident reports serve three purposes:

1. To inform administrators, so that patterns and trends can be monitored. This is called risk management. The goal is to prevent future similar incidents.

2. To alert administrators to possible liability claims.

3. To provide a means of documenting, in a factual manner, information that may be used for detecting possible future problems.

Most employers make incident report forms available to professionals. Forms vary with each facility. However, they usually require the following information:

- The identities of the persons involved and any witnesses
- What happened
- Consequences to the person(s) involved
- Date and time of incident
- Location of incident
- Signature of person making report

Incident report forms should be completed in an objective, factual manner. Incident reports should not include the following types of statements:

- Emotional descriptions of what happened
- Opinions (such as what you think may happen because of the incident)
- Assumptions (what you think caused the incident)
- Finger pointing (who you think was responsible for the incident)

If an incident results from the phlebotomist's own error, the phlebotomist still has the responsibility to file an incident report. It is possible that the phlebotomist's supervisor will take corrective action because of the incident, but a reprimand is likely to be less severe in this case than if the phlebotomist does not report the incident or attempts to cover up the error.

Immediate, factual, and accurate reporting are essential for risk management and quality assurance. In fact, risk management and quality assurance are closely related. Both activities are important for the protection of the patient, the employer, and the health care professional. Phlebotomists need to understand the concepts of risk management and quality assurance so that they may contribute to the well-being of the patient and the employer. Risk management and quality assurance both make use of the information gathered through the reporting system and use the information in the same way, applying the same methodology:

- Identifying a risk or problem
- Monitoring
- Identifying trends
- Summarizing
- Prescribing corrective action
- Evaluating the effectiveness of the correction

The difference between the two areas is that risk management is involved with financial liability issues, while quality assurance seeks to eliminate or reduce patient case problems. The goal of risk management is to avoid risks that could cause financial loss. Quality assurance uses most of the same processes as risk management to assure quality care. Quality assurance is not financially oriented. Both activities are geared toward protection, however. They are intended to protect the patient, the health care worker, and the health care institution through the elimination or reduction of risk.

■ HEALTH CARE FACILITIES THAT UTILIZE PHLEBOTOMISTS

Phlebotomists have the opportunity to work in a variety of health care facilities. Hospitals, clinics, physician offices, nursing homes, blood donor centers, insurance companies, and commercial laboratories all employ phlebotomists. Job duties may vary greatly, but the primary job duty is to collect blood samples.

Hospitals vary in size, the type of care and services provided, and the type of ownership. The size of a hospital is usually described by the number of patient beds in the facility. For instance, a large hospital such as Cedar-Sinai Medical Center in Los Angeles, California, had 952 beds and 55,486 inpatient admissions in 2007. A medium-sized hospital like Baptist Health South Florida in Miami, Florida, had 680 beds and 31,792 admissions in 2008. Penrose-St. Francis Hospital in Colorado Springs, Colorado, also a medium-sized hospital, had 522 beds and 23,258 admissions in 2008. A smaller hospital like Seattle Children's Hospital in Seattle, Washington, had 250 beds with a huge number of outpatient visits (176,608) in 2007.

A phlebotomist may deduce that a large hospital will need a larger phlebotomy staff for inpatient laboratory collections. However, a small hospital such as Seattle Children's Hospital requires a larger staff due not to the size of the hospital but to the number of outpatient visits. Hospitals offer a large variety of services and specialties. Services may include birth centers, cancer centers, critical care, emergency/trauma, pediatric care, rehabilitation services, surgical services, imaging/radiology, cardiovascular programs, neurological services, and many other specialties. For instance, Bellevue Hospital Center in New York City is the oldest public hospital in the United States with 809 beds. It has long been identified with treating mental illness. The University of Texas M.D. Anderson Cancer Center is well known for outstanding cancer treatment and is a 521-bed hospital.

Hospitals are also categorized by their type of ownership. Private hospitals are owned by a corporation and are expected to produce a profit from delivering health services. The profit is returned to the owner or stockholders. A nonprofit hospital may make money, but the money is returned to the organization. Nonprofit hospitals are normally run by a board of directors. Hospitals may also be owned by a state, county, or city government. Taxpayer dollars help fund the operation of the hospital.

Commercial diagnostic laboratories are another type of facility that employs phlebotomists. Commercial laboratories offer testing services for patients referred by their physician. Commercial laboratories such a LabCorp and Quest Diagnostics have large testing facilities with several off-site blood collection stations.

Insurance companies and nursing homes employ phlebotomists who often perform other duties in addition to blood collection. Insurance companies send the phlebotomist to the homes of potential patients to collect blood samples as part of the required health physical. Nursing homes utilize certified nursing assistants with phlebotomy skills to provide care to patients and collect blood specimens for laboratory testing.

■ CLINICAL LABORATORY DEPARTMENTS

Phlebotomy students assigned to a medical laboratory to complete an internship should have a basic knowledge of the departments that comprise the laboratory. Medical laboratory testing plays a crucial role in the detection, diagnosis, and treatment of disease. The laboratory may be divided into two areas of testing: clinical pathology and anatomic pathology. The anatomic pathology laboratory may include histopathology, cytopathology, electron microscopy, and surgical pathology. The clinical pathology laboratory may include chemistry, blood bank, hematology, microbiology, toxicology, immunology, serology, and phlebotomy. The division of departments varies from one facility to another. The pathology laboratory designs the testing departments based upon several factors such as workload, type of tests offered, and other miscellaneous factors. Brief descriptions of the department within the pathology laboratory are as follows:

- Chemistry. May use serum, whole blood, or plasma for testing. The department tests for chemicals present in blood. Lipids, blood sugar, enzymes, and hormones are tested.
- Hematology. Requires whole blood for most tests. Complete blood counts are the most common test. Please refer to Figure 1-4.

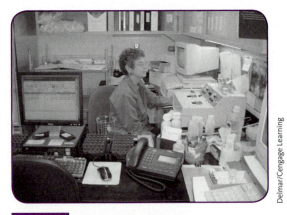

Delmar/Cengage Learning

Figure 1-4 Hematologist at work.

- Microbiology. May use almost any specimen type including feces, urine, blood, sputum, swabs, cerebrospinal fluid, synovial fluid, and tissue. The primary concerns cultures to look for pathogens. Once the pathogen has been determined, a sensitivity test is run to determine the appropriate medication for killing the organism.

- Coagulation. Requires citrated blood. The department is responsible for determining clotting times and coagulation factors.

- Blood Bank. Uses primarily serum and anticoagulated whole blood for testing. The purpose of the department is to provide transfusion medicine. It performs ABO blood Rh typing; prepares blood components, derivatives, and products for transfusion; and may include a section for communication and contact for blood donations.

- Urinalysis. Examines urine for many analytes. The department may be an independent laboratory, or it may be combined with hematology or chemistry.

- **Histopathology.** Processes solid tissue for evaluation at the microscopic level. It requires a variety of staining techniques.

- **Cytopathology.** Examines smears of cells (such as from the cervix) for possible inflammation, cancer, and other conditions. Cells in urine or sputum may be placed in a preservative for examination.

- Cytogenetics. Uses blood and tissue for DNA analysis.

- Surgical Pathology. Examines organs, tumors, fetuses, and other tissues biopsied in surgery.

- Phlebotomy. Consists of specimen collection, specimen processing, point-of-care testing, and clerical functions. Please refer to Figure 1-5 and Figure 1-6.

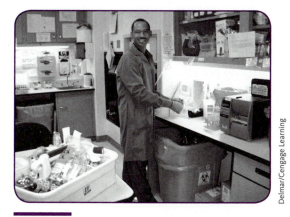

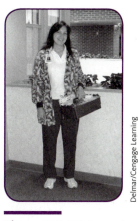

Delmar/Cengage Learning

Figure 1-5 Phlebotomist performing specimen processing duties.

Figure 1-6 Phlebotomist assigned to specimen collection duties.

■ STUDY SKILLS

Good study skills are a very important element in becoming a successful student in the classroom. Adult students may find themselves entering a very exciting and stimulating environment. However, the feelings of excitement and joy may also be accompanied with feelings of anxiety, fear, and stress. Some students may be returning to the classroom after spending years as a stay-at-home mom, or after working many years in a career that has been abruptly ended by downsizing at the company, or even loss of a job due to the company closing its doors. The fear and anxiety comes from the unknown. Will I be able to learn the material? Will I be able to get acceptable grades on exams? Will I be able to compete with other students? Am I too old, too young, too inexperienced? And on and on it goes with the self-doubt and insecurities. The answer to the unknown is to take away as much of the unknown as possible, and put a controlled environment into place. The student should set up an organized, planned study routine that is strictly practiced on a daily basis.

Before the Classroom

The time to begin learning starts with researching schools and career goals. Phlebotomy students should research lab technician/phlebotomy requirements. There are many fine community colleges that offer certificate programs in phlebotomy. There are also many good private schools that offer phlebotomy training. Research the schools that would be available to you. Check courses offered, costs, and time elements that will suit your individual needs. Check job opportunities for phlebotomists and lab technicians, potential pay, and any other factors of concern to you. Once you have decided upon a school, complete a school application. Completing a school application is not difficult and relatively inexpensive. When you have been accepted to the school, make an appointment with a school advisor. The advisor will help you plan courses and schedule any other school requirements. Obtain a school catalogue and read everything about the school as well as your certificate or degree pathway. The more you learn about your school, the more you will be comfortable in your new environment. You will not be faced with the unknown and unpleasant surprises.

The Classroom

Once the student has enrolled in a program, it is very important to prepare for the classroom. The following offers suggestions that will lead to success:

- Have reading and homework assignments completed. Before leaving home for class, take a moment to check for school supplies. Pencils, pens, notebooks, folders, and so on should be in your possession before you enter the classroom. Have your reading assignments completed so that you can participate in class discussions. Highlight important sections in your textbook. Make notes of questions that you may have. Complete all homework assignments. Don't wait until late the evening before class to complete assignments. Unexpected events may prevent you from completing your assignments. Allow yourself time if you have computer or printer malfunctions. Instructors always hear unfortunate stories about "My printer ran out of ink," "My computer was acting up," or "My children were ill." Plan and prepare ahead of class time.

- Be on time for class. Arriving late to class is disruptive. It is disrespectful to your instructor and to your fellow classmates. Arrive slightly early and select a seat that is close to the front. You can hear the instructor better, see the visual aids better, and allow the instructor to get to know you, especially in a large class. Don't sit next to someone who is a distraction. You have paid for the class. Get your money's worth!

- Take notes. Listen to the instructor and outline the lecture as it is presented. Be alert for key ideas and statements. If it is difficult for you to take notes, ask the instructor if you can record the lecture. Review your notes and revise them the same day. Waiting longer to review your notes may result in not knowing what you wrote. A good technique is to put your notes on index cards with different categories. Or type your notes into your computer with categories. Take time to spell key terms correctly. Correct spelling is important in health care. Medical terms may be difficult to spell, but you need to take time to learn them correctly.

- Ask good questions in class. Don't interrupt the instructor. Wait until the instructor asks for questions. It is very disruptive to the class to constantly interject comments or ask questions at inappropriate times. When addressing the instructor or class, speak up so that the entire class can hear your comments and questions. Participate in class discussions. Sitting silently is like a good book sitting on the shelf. If it is not read, it has no value.

- Respect your instructor's time and space. When the instructor arrives in the classroom, give her time to get her personal belongings settled. Ask if this is a good time to talk. Or ask if you could schedule a time to meet. Don't send your instructor unnecessary e-mails or phone calls. There are many students requesting attention. Be considerate and ask necessary questions that cannot be saved until class time.

- Do not bring food and drink to the classroom, unless your instructor has given permission. Rustling snack bags is very disruptive and disrespectful to the instructor and the class. Eating during lecture time is distracting to you. You are not focusing on the lecture if you are eating. Throw away your drink containers and trash. Leaving them on your desk turns your instructor into a housekeeper.

- Review your class syllabus regularly. Be prepared for the topic of the day as well as for future classes.

- Check out your school's study center. Most higher education facilities have study centers where you can get help. Take full advantage of all the services your school has to offer.

- Prepare yourself mentally for a good class. Put aside worries, problems, and so on and allow yourself to enjoy your class time. This is time for you. Be positive and happy, and you will get more out of your class.

Preparing for Exams

Examinations may be a time of anxiety for many students. The following tips for exam preparation may help you to perform at an optimal level when taking an exam.

- Preparing for an exam should begin at the beginning of a course. Review your notes and handouts regularly. Review your reading assignments immediately after reading. Study difficult material until you feel comfortable with it. Do not wait until the day before an exam to study. You will have a difficult time absorbing the material.

- Study in blocks of 30–60 minutes. Take short breaks. Study without distractions, in a quiet place. Television and music will not allow you to focus.

- Plan a schedule. Block out specific time for studying. Ask family members not to disturb you during your scheduled study time. Be disciplined. Don't look for excuses to delay your study time.

Taking the Exam

Once you have prepared for the exam, the following tips will help in taking it:

- Get sufficient sleep. Do not stay up late cramming. Eat a light breakfast or snack.
- Arrive on time. Arriving late for an exam decreases your exam time, and causes you to be unfocused.
- Make sure you have all necessary supplies such as pens, pencils, paper, and so on.
- Look over the exam and have a basic plan for how much time to spend on each section. Answer the easier sections first. Save the difficult sections for last so that you have more time to focus.
- Put your name and date on the exam. It is not unusual for students to forget to place this information on the exam. Place all notebooks, textbooks, and paper off of your desk.
- Read the questions thoroughly and carefully. Do not assume anything. Ask for clarification, if necessary.
- If you are unsure of an answer, do not leave the question unanswered. Make a good guess.
- Watch the clock. Do not allow yourself to run out of time.
- When you have completed the exam, review it. Make sure you have answered all questions. Turn your exam in to the instructor, and do not disrupt other students.

CLINICAL ASSIGNMENT EXPECTATIONS

Many phlebotomy training programs involve a lecture section combined with an internship section. The internship is basically an on-the-job training period that allows the student to apply skills learned in the classroom to real life situations involving patients and medical staff. The clinical internship allows for many opportunities in networking with medical professionals, learning an appreciation of the stresses and rewards of the medical field, and building lifelong memories and knowledge. The rewards come with several responsibilities:

- Arrive on time at your assigned health care facility. One of the most important aspects of a phlebotomist's duties is to draw specimens in a timely manner. Stat, ASAP, and timed collections must be drawn at the appropriate time.

- Maintain a professional appearance. Early **morning rounds** may start as early as 3:00 A.M. Go to bed early enough the previous evening so that you are rested and energized. Allow yourself enough time to be well groomed for the performance of your duties. Look your best every day. Follow the health care facility's dress code. A good appearance will give you confidence and increase your self-esteem.

- Maintain a well-stocked and organized phlebotomy collection tray. Your tray or cart represents your work area, and is a reflection of the quality of your work.

- Ensure appropriate, timely, and professional communication with patients, staff, and physicians. Your attention should be on the patient and your assigned duties. Do not discuss personal issues such as financial concerns, family problems, your opinions about medical care, etc., with the patient. Do not have disagreements or arguments with staff in front of the patient. Be courteous and respectful at all times with everyone in the internship environment.

- Ask good questions and show a keen interest in your work. Do not challenge the health care staff about the correctness of procedures. If you see something that seems wrong or inappropriate, direct your concerns to your instructor. Remember that you are a guest at the facility. Thank the staff for the information and help that has been given to you.

- Introduce yourself to supervisors and other staff. You may wish to seek employment with the facility after your internship. The job market is very competitive, and forming a favorable impression with health care professionals at your internship site may be very helpful in your job search.

■ SUMMARY

The role of the student carries with it both responsibilities and rewards. As you begin to learn your role, keep the following thoughts in mind:

- Learn the procedures and protocols of your profession accurately.
- Interact with all members of your health care team in a positive and professional manner.

- Know your instructors' expectations. Respect your fellow students and your instructors by practicing good classroom etiquette.
- Know and appreciate the history of your profession.
- Maintain goals to expand your medical knowledge each day. Enjoy your patients and your role in providing them with quality health care.

▨ REVIEW ACTIVITIES

1. The two primary job duties of a laboratory phlebotomist are:

   a. _____

   b. _____

2. A phlebotomist collects blood samples by using three techniques:

   a. _____

   b. _____

   c. _____

3. List five types of patients who will interact with the phlebotomist.

   a. _____

   b. _____

   c. _____

   d. _____

   e. _____

4. Phlebotomists should not gossip with patients about fellow workers or physicians because _____.

5. Phlebotomists should not encourage patients to ask for a specific "favorite" phlebotomist to draw specimens because _____.

6. A bill of rights for patients is designed to _____ _____.

7. _____ is a system that examines values, actions, and choices to determine right and wrong.

8. _____ are strongly held personal and professional beliefs.

9. _____ is a method of monitoring the quality of patient care.

10. The five techniques used for bloodletting in the past were _____, _____, _____, _____, and _____.

11. Galen believed that the arteries in the body contained _____.

12. Realdus Columbus discovered the _____ circulation.

13. _____ is credited with our modern understanding of the circulatory system.

14. The _____ was the early version of the phlebotomist.

15. HIPAA is the first comprehensive federal protection law for the privacy of _____ _____.

16. An anatomic pathology laboratory may include _____, _____, _____, and _____.

17. The clinical pathology laboratory may include _____, _____, _____, _____, _____, _____, and _____.

18. Preparing for an exam should begin _____.

19. When working as an intern, any disagreements with a staff member should be directed to your _____.

■ DISCUSSION QUESTIONS

1. You go into a patient's room to draw a blood sample. The patient's physician is present. You ask the physician if you should return or draw the blood sample now. The physician indicates that she wants you to draw the blood now. When you introduce yourself to the patient, he says that he does not want his blood drawn. The physician explains to the patient that test results are necessary for her to determine further treatment. The patient is adamant, and refuses. The physician tells you to draw the blood. What should you do?

2. You are drawing a patient's blood in the outpatient laboratory. When you have completed the collection, you thank the patient and raise the drawing chair arm so that the patient may leave. The patient stands, faints, and suddenly falls to the floor. After the patient has been revived, it is determined that he has sustained a bump on the head. The patient refuses to be taken to the emergency department or to be seen by a physician. He insists that he is fine, and leaves the outpatient lab. What should you do?

2

The Student's Role in the Clinical Environment

OBJECTIVES

After studying this unit, it is the responsibility of the learner to be able to:

1. Describe OSHA's role as a federal agency.
2. Describe the standard precautions system.
3. State the five major tactics OSHA has developed to reduce the risk of exposure to bloodborne pathogens.
4. Demonstrate proper hand-washing technique.
5. Describe the procedure for proper sharps disposal.
6. State the requirements for wearing gloves.
7. Demonstrate the appropriate glove removal procedure.
8. List the general rules for housekeeping for the phlebotomist.
9. Discuss the chemical, electrical, and radiation hazards that a phlebotomist might encounter.

KEY TERMS

bloodborne pathogens pathogenic microorganisms that can be present in blood and can cause disease

CAP College of American Pathologists, a medical society comprised exclusively of pathologists serving over 15,000 physician members and the laboratory community worldwide that is widely considered the leader in providing laboratory quality improvement programs

CDC The Centers for Disease Control and Prevention, an agency of the Department of Health and Human Services. Its function is to promote health and quality of life by preventing and controlling disease, injury, and disability

CLSI Clinical Laboratory Standards Institute (formerly NCCLS), an institute that sets standards for specimen collection and handling to protect the patient from injury and negative outcomes

contaminated referring to the presence of blood or infectious material on an item or surface

decontaminate the use of physical or chemical means to destroy bloodborne pathogens on a surface to the point where they are no longer able to transmit infectious particles

engineering controls controls such as sharps disposal and the use of containers and self-sheathing needles, which isolate or remove a bloodborne pathogens hazard

HBV hepatitis B virus

HCV hepatitis C virus

HICPAC Healthcare Infection Control Practices Advisory Committee, a committee consisting of eleven public members and one federal member. Members are selected by the secretary of the DHHS from experts in the fields of infectious diseases, nosocomial infections, nursing, epidemiology, public health, and related areas of expertise. One of the primary functions of the committee is to issue recommendations for preventing and controlling nosocomial infections in the form of guidelines, resolutions, and informal communications

HIV human immunodeficiency virus

The Joint Commission (formerly known as JCAHO) Joint Commission on Accreditation of Healthcare Organizations, and still commonly referred to as "JCAHO" ("Jay-Co"); an independent, not-for-profit organization that evaluates and accredits health care organizations in the United States

latex allergy an allergic reaction that can result from repeated exposures to proteins in natural rubber latex through skin contact or inhalation

Needlestick Safety and Prevention Act a bill signed November 6, 2000, that contains an amendment to OSHA's bloodborne pathogen standard to ensure more widespread use of safer medical devices to prevent dangerous needlesticks. The legislation requires employers to identify and provide safer equipment for their staffs

NIOSH The National Institute for Occupational Safety and Health, a federal agency responsible for conducting research and making recommendations for the prevention of work-related disease and injury. It is part of the Centers for Disease Control and Prevention

nosocomial a disorder associated with being treated in a hospital, but unrelated to the patient's primary condition

OSHA Occupational Safety and Health Administration, a federal agency that develops and promotes occupational safety and health standards, develops and issues regulations, conducts investigations and inspections, and issues citations and proposes penalties for noncompliance with safety and health standards and regulations

personal protective equipment (PPE) specialized clothing or equipment worn by a professional for protection against a hazard

sharp an object that can penetrate the skin such as a needle, scalpel, broken glass, broken capillary tube, or lancet

sterilize to use a physical or chemical procedure to destroy all microbial life

universal body substance precautions (UBSP) an approach to infection control that considers all human blood and certain body fluids to be infectious and handles them as such

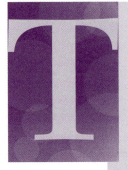he health care environment can be a dangerous place, both for the phlebotomist and for the patient. Providing excellent care in a safe environment must be the foremost concern for health care providers. There are biological, chemical, electrical, and radiation dangers that must be understood by the phlebotomist, so that such hazards can be eliminated or minimized. Many regulatory and professional agencies—such as the Occupational Safety and Health Administration (**OSHA**), the College of American Pathologists (**CAP**), Clinical Laboratory Standards Institute (CLSI), The Joint Commission (formerly known as **JCAHO**), the Centers for Disease Control and Prevention (**CDC**), the National Institute for Occupational Safety and Health (**NIOSH**), and the Healthcare Infection Control Practices Advisory Committee (**HICPAC**)—recognize the need to ensure health and safety standards for the health professional.

■ OSHA

OSHA is a federal agency that was established as a result of the Occupational Safety and Health Act of 1970. The agency works to promote safety in the health care environment in these ways:

- Developing and promoting occupational safety and health standards
- Developing and issuing regulations
- Conducting investigations and inspections to determine the status of compliance with safety and health standards and regulations
- Issuing citations and proposing penalties for noncompliance with safety and health standards and regulations

OSHA's concern is for the worker. Patient safety and health is not under its jurisdiction. OSHA has developed a set of health and safety standards for the protection of the health care worker entitled *Occupational Exposure to Bloodborne Pathogens Final Rule 1910.1030*. Every health care facility should have an exposure control plan developed in accordance with the OSHA standards. Phlebotomists should read and understand their facility's exposure plan. The OSHA standards detail ways to reduce the risk of contracting a bloodborne disease while on the job.

The **College of American Pathologists (CAP)** is a medical society comprised exclusively of pathologists serving over 15,000 physician members and the laboratory community worldwide. It is widely considered the leader in providing laboratory quality improvement programs. CAP reviews safety practices and policies such as fire drills, chemical hygiene plans, safe handling of electrical equipment, proper use of personal protective clothing and equipment, policies for prohibiting recapping and bending of needles, and policies for infection control that comply with the OSHA standard on occupational exposure to **bloodborne pathogens**.

The **Centers for Disease Control and Prevention (CDC)** is an agency of the Department of Health and Human Services. Its function is to promote health and quality of life by preventing and controlling disease, injury, and disability. The CDC includes eleven centers:

Office of the Director
Epidemiology Programs
National Center for Chronic Disease Prevention and Health
    Promotion
National Center for Environmental Health, Genetics, and Disease
    Prevention
National Center for Health Statistics
National Center for HIV, STD, and TB Prevention
National Center for Infectious Diseases
National Center for Injury Prevention and Control
National Immunization Program
National Institute for Occupational Safety and Health
Public Health Practice Program Office

The **National Institute for Occupational Safety and Health (NIOSH)** is the federal agency responsible for conducting research and making recommendations for the prevention of work-related disease and injury. It is part of the CDC. NIOSH was established by the Occupational Safety and Health Act of 1970. That act also established OSHA. While NIOSH and OSHA were created by the same act of Congress, they are different agencies with separate responsibilities. NIOSH is in the Department of Health and Human Services and is a research agency. OSHA is in the Department of Labor and is responsible for creating and enforcing workplace safety and health regulations.

The **National Committee for Clinical Laboratories Standards (NCCLS)** is a nonprofit standards-developing and educational organization that promotes the development and use of voluntary consensus standards and guidelines within the health care community.

The **Clinical and Laboratory Standards Institute** (CLSI, formerly NCCLS) sets standards for specimen collection, handling, and testing to protect the patient from injury and negative outcomes. The goal of the institute is to help laboratories maintain a high level of performance required to pass various inspections.

The Joint Commission (formerly known as JCAHO) is a not-for-profit accrediting body. It accredits approximately 20,000 health care organizations and programs each year in the United States. The Joint Commission (formerly known as JCAHO) has been in operation since 1951, developing professional-based standards and evaluating compliance of health care organizations against those standards. Accreditation is recognized as a symbol of quality that indicates an organization meets certain performance standards.

BIOLOGICAL HAZARDS AND STANDARD PRECAUTIONS

Phlebotomists must always use great care in handling biological substances such as blood, urine, and other materials collected from the human body. Because needles are a primary tool utilized by the phlebotomist, a special emphasis must be placed on efforts to guard against exposure—of the worker and the patient—to bloodborne diseases. Between 800,000 and 1,000,000 accidental needlesticks are reported in the United States each year. Exposure may also occur through open cuts or abrasions and contact of the eye, nose, or mouth with the patient's blood. As reported in the "Pilot Study of Needlestick Prevention Devices," there are more than 20 pathogens transmitted by needlesticks. The most serious are hepatitis C (**HCV**), hepatitis B (**HBV**), and **HIV**. Although there are few documented cases of AIDS due to occupational exposure, OSHA reports that approximately 8,700 health care workers each year contract HBV. About 200 will die as a result. In addition, some who become carriers will pass the disease on to others. Carriers also face a higher risk for liver ailments, including cirrhosis of the liver and primary liver cancer.

OSHA makes use of the **universal body substance precautions (UBSP)**, now referred to as standard precautions system, in its standards (see Figure 2-1). The system is interaction-driven, meaning it assumes that *all* blood and *all* bodily substances of *all* patients are potentially infectious. In the past, the isolation system was used, which was based on the patient's diagnosis. Since it is impossible to know the status of all patients' blood for HBV, HIV, and other infectious diseases, the UBSP system is much more appropriate for reducing risks to the health care worker.

STANDARD PRECAUTIONS

Assume that every person is potentially infected or colonized with an organism that could be transmitted in the healthcare setting.

Hand Hygiene

Avoid unnecessary touching of surfaces in close proximity to the patient.

When hands are visibly dirty, contaminated with proteinaceous material, or visibly soiled with blood or body fluids, wash hands with soap and water.

If hands are not visibly soiled, or after removing visible material with soap and water, decontaminate hands with an alcohol-based hand rub. Alternatively, hands may be washed with an antimicrobial soap and water.

Perform hand hygiene:
Before having direct contact with patients.
After contact with blood, body fluids or excretions, mucous membranes, nonintact skin, or wound dressings.
After contact with a patient's intact skin (e.g., when taking a pulse or blood pressure or lifting a patient).
If hands will be moving from a contaminated-body site to a clean-body site during patient care.
After contact with inanimate objects (including medical equipment) in the immediate vicinity of the patient.
After removing gloves.

Personal protective equipment (PPE)

Wear PPE when the nature of the anticipated patient interaction indicates that contact with blood or body fluids may occur.

Before leaving the patient's room or cubicle, remove and discard PPE.

Gloves

Wear gloves when contact with blood or other potentially infectious materials, mucous membranes, nonintact skin, or potentially contaminated intact skin (e.g., of a patient incontinent of stool or urine) could occur.

Remove gloves after contact with a patient and/or the surrounding environment using proper technique to prevent hand contamination. Do not wear the same pair of gloves for the care of more than one patient.

Change gloves during patient care if the hands will move from a contaminated body-site (e.g., perineal area) to a clean body-site (e.g., face).

Gowns

Wear a gown to protect skin and prevent soiling or contamination of clothing during procedures and patient-care activities when contact with blood, body fluids, secretions, or excretions is anticipated.

Wear a gown for direct patient contact if the patient has uncontained secretions or excretions.

Remove gown and perform hand hygiene before leaving the patient's environment.

Mouth, nose, eye protection

Use PPE to protect the mucous membranes of the eyes, nose and mouth during procedures and patient-care activities that are likely to generate splashes or sprays of blood, body fluids, secretions and excretions.

During aerosol-generating procedures wear one of the following: a face shield that fully covers the front and sides of the face, a mask with attached shield, or a mask and goggles.

Respiratory Hygiene/Cough Etiquette

Educate healthcare personnel to contain respiratory secretions to prevent droplet and fomite transmission of respiratory pathogens, especially during seasonal outbreaks of viral respiratory tract infections.

Offer masks to coughing patients and other symptomatic persons (e.g., persons who accompany ill patients) upon entry into the facility.

Patient-care equipment and instruments/devices

Wear PPE (e.g., gloves, gown), according to the level of anticipated contamination, when handling patient-care equipment and instruments/devices that are visibly soiled or may have been in contact with blood or body fluids.

Care of the environment

Include multi-use electronic equipment in policies and procedures for preventing contamination and for cleaning and disinfection, especially those items that are used by patients, those used during delivery of patient care, and mobile devices that are moved in and out of patient rooms frequently (e.g., daily).

Textiles and laundry

Handle used textiles and fabrics with minimum agitation to avoid contamination of air, surfaces and persons.

SPR   ©2007 Brevis Corporation www.brevis.com

Reprinted with permission from Brevis Corporation (www.brevis.com)

Figure 2-1 Standard precautions.

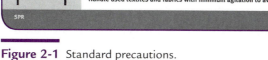

OSHA has developed five major methods to reduce the risk of exposure to bloodborne pathogens:

1. Engineering controls
2. Work practices
3. Personal protective equipment
4. Housekeeping
5. Hepatitis B vaccination

Engineering Controls

There are physical and mechanical devices on the market designed to reduce or eliminate the hazard of transferring potentially infectious diseases. Some examples of these **engineering controls** include self-sheathing needles, vented safety hoods (also called biosafety cabinets) where infectious materials can be handled, autoclaves that **sterilize** the **contaminated** materials, and hard plastic specimen disposal units.

The **Needlestick Safety and Prevention Act** was signed November 6, 2000, to further ensure usage of safer medical devices. Because each year one in seven medical professionals experiences a needlestick while caring for sick or injured patients, it is essential that employers provide safer equipment to help prevent many of these injuries. In March 2000, the CDC estimated that more than 380,000 percutaneous injuries from contaminated **sharps** occur annually among health care workers in U.S. hospital settings. Numerous studies have demonstrated that the use of safer medical devices, such as sharps with engineered sharps injury protections, when they are part of an overall bloodborne pathogens risk reduction program, can be extremely effective in reducing needlesticks. The CDC estimates that 62–88 percent of sharps injuries can potentially be prevented by the use of safer medical devices.

A variety of self-sheathing needles are available. A quality product should have these properties:

1. Provide a barrier between the needle and hand after the venipuncture is completed
2. Be relatively easy to operate
3. Allow the phlebotomist's hand/fingers to be behind the needle at all times
4. Ensure that the safety feature be in effect before and after the venipuncture
5. Not interfere with the delivery of the venipuncture during the patient/phlebotomist interaction

Specimen collection tubes are also an example of possible engineering controls. Tubes are available in both plastic and glass. The plastic tubes help to ensure a safer environment should breakage of the tube occur. NIOSH and the Food and Drug Administration suggest that glass capillary tubes not be used. Glass capillary tubes have broken when inserted into putty to be sealed, and during centrifugation. The joint safety advisory recommends:

1. Capillary tubes that are not made of glass
2. Glass capillary tubes wrapped in puncture-resistant film
3. Products that use a method of sealing that does not require manually pushing one end of the tube into putty to form a plug
4. Products that allow blood cells to be measured without centrifugation

Specimen containers should be transported in sealed plastic bags. Requisitions should not be placed inside the bag with the specimen.

Sharps containers are another engineering control. Containers for sharps must be puncture-resistant. The sides and the bottom must be leak proof. They must be labeled or color-coded red to ensure that everyone knows the contents are hazardous. Containers must have a lid, and they must be maintained upright to keep liquids and the sharps inside. Containers must be properly disposed of when two-thirds full. Please refer to Figure 2-2.

Phlebotomists must never reach by hand into containers of contaminated sharps. Once closed, containers are never to be reopened or

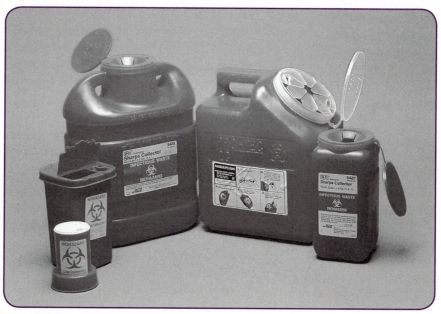

Delmar/Cengage Learning

Figure 2-2 Puncture-proof sharps container.

emptied into another container. As many as one-third of all sharps injuries have been reported to be related to the disposal process. The U.S. Department of Health and Human Services states that disposal injuries occur because of the following:

1. Inadequate design or inappropriate placement of the sharps disposal container
2. Overfilling of sharps disposal containers
3. Inappropriate sharps disposal practices by the user during patient care

Correctly and consistently using physical and mechanical devices designed for the phlebotomist's safety will help to reduce and possibly eliminate injuries.

Work Practices

NIOSH recommends that health care workers take the following steps to protect themselves and their coworkers from needlestick injuries:

1. Help your employer select and evaluate devices with safety features.
2. Use devices with safety features provided by your employer. Immediately activate the safety feature once the blood sample is collected.
3. Do not recap needles. OSHA allows recapping "when no alternative is feasible." If recapping of a needle takes place, the manager must justify the practice in the exposure control manual and support the practice with documented evidence.
4. Transfer devices should be used when transferring blood from a syringe into collection tubes. Do not transfer by puncturing the rubber stopper of the collection tube with a needle attached to the syringe.
5. Tube holders are not to be reused. In 2003 OSHA issued a bulletin stating, "OSHA has concluded that the best practice for prevention of needlestick injuries following phlebotomy procedures is the use of a sharp with engineered sharps injury protection attached to the blood tube holder and the immediate disposal of the entire unit after each patient's blood is drawn."
6. Plan for safe handling and disposal before beginning any procedure using needles.
7. Dispose of used needles promptly in appropriate sharps disposal containers.

8. Report all needlestick and other sharps-related injuries promptly to ensure that you receive appropriate follow-up care.

9. Tell your employer about hazards from needles that you observe in your work environment.

10. Participate in bloodborne pathogen training and follow recommended infection prevention practices, including hepatitis B vaccination.

Hand washing has been identified as the single most important means of preventing the spread of **nosocomial** infections. The purpose of hand washing is to remove dirt, organic material, and transient microorganisms. Each time phlebotomists remove their gloves they must wash their hands with soap and running water. Gloves must be changed after each patient contact. Should hand-washing facilities not be immediately available, antiseptic hand cleanser or antiseptic towelettes must be used. These are temporary measures, however, and hands must be washed with soap and running water as soon as possible.

PROCEDURE   Hand Washing

1. Remove rings from fingers. If a watch is worn, move it above wrist level or remove it.

2. Adjust the water to a warm temperature, and allow it to continue running.

3. Wet the hands (see Figure 2-3).

4. Apply soap and lather thoroughly. The friction from rubbing hands is very important for removing potentially infectious organisms (see Figure 2-4). Lather vigorously for at least 10 seconds.

5. Clean under nails and around nail beds with the nails of the opposite hand (see Figure 2-5). A nail brush may be used if available.

6. Thoroughly rinse each hand from the wrist down.

7. Dry hands with disposable towels.

8. Turn off the faucet with a used towel (see Figure 2-6). The towel will protect the hands from the contaminated faucet handle.

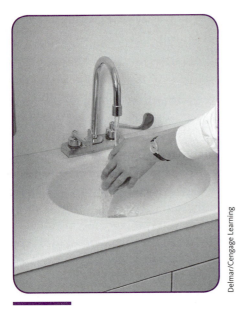

Figure 2-3 Wet the hands.

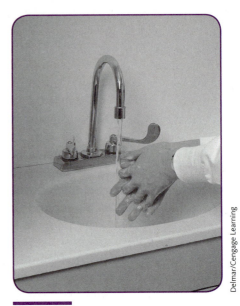

Figure 2-4 The friction from rubbing hands is very important for removing potentially infectious organisms.

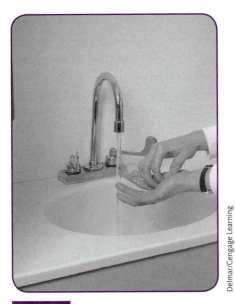

Figure 2-5 Clean under nails and around nail beds with the nails of the opposite hand.

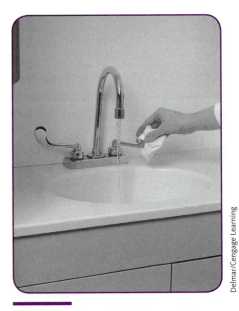

Figure 2-6 Turn off the faucet with a used towel.

PROCEDURE   One-Handed Recapping Method

To be used only when manager has written a protocol in the exposure control plan.

1. Place needle cap on a flat surface. This prevents the cap from rolling away.

2. Position the needle unit on the same plane as the cap, aligning the needle and cap.

3. Scoop up the cap with the needle unit. Scooping with one hand prevents accidental needle puncture of the opposite hand.

4. Press the cap on the flat surface to secure the cap to the needle unit. Using the surface instead of the opposite hand prevents accidental needle punctures.

5. Dispose of the recapped needle. All sharps must *always* be disposed of immediately to prevent the possibility of an accidental needle puncture. Additional work practice controls include the following:

   · Eating, drinking, smoking, applying cosmetics or lip balm, and handling contact lenses are not allowed in work areas where exposure to potentially infectious materials may occur.

   · Food and drink are not to be kept in areas where potentially infectious materials are present.

   · Never mouth a pipette.

   · Take every precaution to minimize splashes or spraying when performing procedures involving potentially infectious materials. Commercial products such as goggles, face shields, and splash screens may be used.

Personal Protective Equipment

Protective equipment used by the phlebotomist may include gloves, masks, gowns, lab coats, face shields, goggles, and mouthpieces. The purpose of such **personal protective equipment (PPE)** is to prevent potentially infectious material from contacting work clothes, street clothes, skin, or mucous membranes. The type of equipment used depends on the degree of exposure anticipated. The phlebotomist's job requires exposure to bloodborne pathogens. Therefore employers must provide the appropriate protective equipment at no cost. In addition, the equipment must be cleaned, laundered, repaired, replaced, or disposed of at no cost to the professional.

The employer and the phlebotomist must work as a team to comply with OSHA requirements. The phlebotomist must be trained to use the equipment properly. It is particularly important that gloves fit properly. A variety of sizes must be made available. In addition, hypoallergenic gloves, glove liners, or powderless gloves must be made available for those allergic to latex or nylon gloves.

Gloves are the most frequently used form of personal protective equipment. The phlebotomist must wear gloves when contact with blood, potentially infectious material, mucous membranes, or nonnintact skin is anticipated. This means that phlebotomists must wear gloves for all specimen collection procedures. Bandage any cuts before putting on gloves. Disposable gloves are to be replaced as soon as possible if they become contaminated or damaged in any way. Disposable gloves are never to be washed for reuse. Responsible phlebotomists often put on new gloves in the presence of a patient. Otherwise, patients may be concerned that gloves have been worn in previous patient contacts.

PROCEDURE   Removal of Gloves

1. With one hand, hook a finger in the opposite hand's glove at the outside surface of the opening of the glove (see Figure 2-7). This action prevents the contaminated glove from touching the inside surface of the glove and the skin.

2. Pull the glove off the hand, thus turning the glove inside out (see Figure 2-8). The contaminated surface will be on the inside.

3. Hold the removed glove in the gloved hand. This way you avoid placing the contaminated glove on a clean surface.

4. Hook a finger of the ungloved hand on the *inside* of the remaining glove (see Figure 2-9). The skin does not touch the contaminated outside surface of the glove.

5. Pull the glove off the hand, turning it inside out.

6. Discard gloves immediately in a designated waste container (see Figure 2-10). All contaminated materials must be disposed

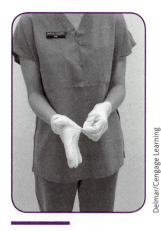

Figure 2-7 With one hand, hook a finger in the opposite hand's glove at the outside surface of the opening of the glove.

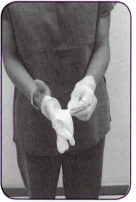

Figure 2-8 Pull the glove off the hand, thus turning the glove inside out.

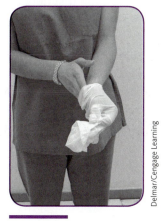

Figure 2-9 Hook a finger of the ungloved hand on the *inside* of the remaining glove.

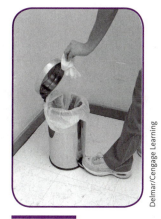

Figure 2-10 Discard gloves immediately in a designated waste container.

of immediately to prevent potential exposure of patients and coworkers.

7. Wash hands. There is always the possibility that there are small holes in gloves.

Gowns are to be worn when the phlebotomist is likely to soil clothes with potentially infectious secretions or excretions. Masks are worn to prevent transmission of airborne infectious agents, and during procedures that are likely to create droplets of blood or other bodily substances. Masks must be changed between each patient contact and discarded in appropriate disposal receptacles after use. Masks must never be reused. Masks should fit snugly over the nose and mouth. Remove the mask by holding the tie at the back of the head. Do not touch the front of the mask. Dispose of used masks in a designated container.

Housekeeping

Good housekeeping is the responsibility of all health care workers. Each health care facility has a control plan that specifies housekeeping requirements. General rules for housekeeping include:

- Clean and **decontaminate** all equipment and work surfaces at the end of each shift. Immediately clean and decontaminate all spills of blood and other bodily fluids. Chemical germicides that are approved for use as hospital disinfectants and are tuberculocidal (able to kill tuberculosis bacilli) when used at recommended dilutions can be used to decontaminate potentially infectious spills. Gloves must be worn while cleaning.
- Do not use gloved or bare hands to pick up broken glass that may be contaminated with infectious material. Use a brush and a dustpan or other devices, such as tongs or forceps.
- Place sharps and infectious waste in designated containers. Sharps containers should never be filled more than 80 percent full.
- Handle contaminated protective clothing as little as possible. Place in labeled containers for laundering.
- Be familiar with the biohazard sign that warns when containers hold blood or other potentially infectious materials (see Figure 2-11).

Hepatitis B Vaccination

Hepatitis B vaccine must be made available at no charge to health care workers who at any time may be exposed to blood or bodily fluids. The vaccine is administered in three injections over a period of six months. The completed series of vaccinations is very effective—for nine years or longer—in protecting the phlebotomist from contracting the disease or becoming a carrier. The phlebotomist should immediately report any defined exposure to the employer. Blood or bodily fluid can come in contact with the phlebotomist via a needlestick, a cut, or a splash to

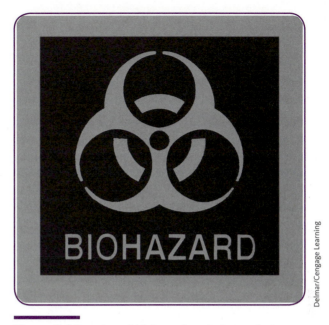

Delmar/Cengage Learning

Figure 2-11 Universal biohazard symbol. *See color insert.*

the eye, nose, or mouth, or through chapped, abraded, or dermatitis-affected skin.

It is the responsibility of phlebotomists to protect themselves from bloodborne pathogens by knowing their employer's control plan and taking proper precautions. Phlebotomists, coworkers, and employers can work together as a team to ensure an environment with minimal risks.

■ LATEX ALLERGIES

Latex gloves have proven effective in preventing transmission of many infectious diseases. But for some phlebotomists, exposure to latex may result in skin rashes, hives, itching, and asthma, as well as nasal, eye, and sinus symptoms and, perhaps on a rare occasion, shock.

Natural rubber latex is a processed milky plant product derived from the *Hevea braziliensis* tree found in Southeast Asia and Africa. Several chemicals are added to this fluid during the processing and manufacture of commercial latex. It is the proteins in the latex as well as the added chemicals that cause a range of mild to severe allergic reactions. Some phlebotomists have specific antibodies, called IgE antibodies, which make them hypersensitive to the proteins in natural rubber latex. IgE-mediated reactions to latex proteins are responsible for most of the allergic reactions.

Phlebotomists are at risk for developing **latex allergy**, because they use latex gloves frequently. The most common reaction to latex is irritant contact dermatitis, which is the development of dry, itchy, irritated areas on the hands. The reaction can also result from repeated hand washing and drying, incomplete hand drying, or exposure to powders added to the inside of the gloves. The proteins responsible for latex allergies fasten to powder that is used on some latex gloves. When powdered gloves are worn, more latex protein reaches the skin. Also, when gloves are changed, latex protein powder particles get into the air where they can be inhaled. Some of the products containing latex to which a phlebotomist may be exposed are:

- Blood pressure cuffs
- Disposable gloves
- Tourniquets
- Syringes
- Goggles
- Tops of blood collection tubes

A phlebotomist who has become allergic to latex should take special precautions. Certain medications may reduce the symptoms, but complete latex avoidance is the most effective approach. Many employers are taking steps to provide a latex-free environment for their workers. Non-latex gloves are provided, and should be used by those with latex allergy. Coworkers should not use powdered gloves in the presence of allergic professionals. Phlebotomists should be aware that topical treatments used to relieve symptoms may compromise the barrier function of gloves. Care should be taken in the choice of treatments to relieve contact dermatitis. The allergic reaction should be reported to the employee health nurse, where it will be appropriately documented and treated.

■ CHEMICAL SAFETY

The phlebotomist may come in contact with hazardous chemicals while using cleaning products, when adding preservatives to 24-hour urine containers (different kinds of preservatives, including acids, may be added to the containers), or when transporting specimens to the laboratory. It is always important to remember that water is never added to acid, because a possible reaction may cause splashing.

[ALERT]

Material safety data sheets (MSDS) within the department allow the phlebotomist to check for safety precautions concerning hazardous ingredients in supplies. MSDS contain such information about the manufacturer, product identification, hazardous ingredients, special protection information, and first aid procedures.

Always read container labels before using a product. OSHA requires that hazardous materials be labeled as to the danger of the substance. Substances are labeled as toxic, flammable, or combustible. In the event of a spill or other exposure, consult the first aid measures listed in the laboratory safety manual.

The phlebotomist should know the location of safety showers and eye wash stations and be instructed in their use in order to be prepared for a possible chemical splash or spill. The body part affected should be flushed with water for a minimum of 15 minutes, and this washing should be followed by a visit to the emergency room.

ELECTRICAL SAFETY

Many accidents, such as fires and electrical shocks, can result from using electrical equipment in the laboratory environment. Follow these guidelines for ensuring electrical safety:

- Avoid using extension cords.
- Inspect cords and plugs for fraying and breaks.
- Do not overload electrical circuits.
- Unplug equipment while servicing it. Also unplug equipment that has had liquid spilled on it. Do not plug it in again until the spill is cleaned up and the wiring is dry.
- Discontinue using and unplug malfunctioning equipment.
- Save electrical repairs for trained professionals.

All phlebotomists should know where the fire extinguishers are located in their department and be familiar with their use. They should know how to use fire blankets or heavy toweling to smother fires on clothing. They should also be familiar with the locations of all emergency exits, and know the facility extension to call in case of fire.

■ RADIATION SAFETY

The phlebotomist may encounter radiation hazards when collecting specimens from patients who have had radioactive treatments, when collecting specimens from patients in the radiology department, and when delivering specimens to departments in the laboratory that use radioactive elements in testing.

Radiation exposure depends on the amount of radiation experienced, how far away one is from the source of radioactivity, how long the exposure lasts, and what protective equipment is worn during the exposure. Radiation effects are cumulative. Phlebotomists generally do not receive enough exposure to cause any problems, but they must always be cautious when entering areas displaying the radiation hazard symbol. Please refer to Figure 2-12.

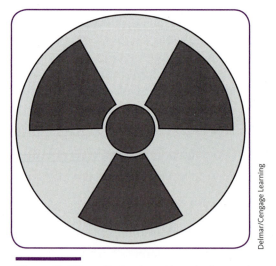

Delmar/Cengage Learning

Figure 2-12 Radiation hazard symbol. *See color insert.*

■ SUMMARY

The phlebotomist must always be vigilant regarding personal and patient safety. The greatest risk to the phlebotomist in the health care environment is exposure to bloodborne pathogens. Hepatitis B is a particular danger, often contracted through needlesticks. Today's health care environment is made safer by the availability of hepatitis B vaccinations. Contracting bloodborne pathogens such as hepatitis, HIV, malaria, and syphilis can be avoided by following procedures set up to minimize such risks.

There are also chemical, electrical, and radiation hazards in the health care environment. Consistently careful work habits should minimize or eliminate most health risks to both the phlebotomist and the patient.

■ REVIEW ACTIVITIES

1. OSHA's concern is for the safety of the _____.

2. _____ and _____ are the two most significant bloodborne diseases encountered by the health care professional.

3. Pathogens may enter the phlebotomist's body through:

   a. _____

   b. _____

4. The standard precautions system is interaction-driven. "Interaction-driven" means _____.

5. OSHA has developed five major methods to reduce risk of exposure to bloodborne pathogens. They are:

   a. _____

   b. _____

   c. _____

   d. _____

   e. _____

6. _____ has been identified as the single most important means of preventing the spread of infection.

7. If needles must be recapped, the appropriate method of recapping is _____.

8. Give five examples of personal protective equipment.

a. _____

b. _____

c. _____

d. _____

e. _____

9. Phlebotomists must wear gloves when _____
_____.

10. The hepatitis B vaccination is administered for the purpose
of _____.

11. Name one duty that phlebotomists may perform that can cause
a chemical burn. _____
_____.

12. Name two electrical safety precautions a phlebotomist can take.

a. _____

b. _____

13. Name two areas where a phlebotomist may come in contact with
radiation hazards.

a. _____

b. _____

■ DISCUSSION QUESTIONS

1. You have just completed drawing blood at the patient's bedside.
You label the collection tubes and are about to bag the tubes for
transport. You knock your collection tray to the floor, spilling
all of the contents as well as breaking the glass tubes of blood
you just collected. What steps should be taken to rectify the
situation?

2. You have accidentally stuck yourself with a contaminated needle.
What steps should you take?

Blood and Urine Collection

3

The Circulatory System

OBJECTIVES

After studying this unit, it is the responsibility of the learner to be able to:

1. Describe the flow of blood through the heart.
2. Describe the branching of the artery network.
3. Describe the venous system of the arm.
4. Explain the components of plasma.
5. State the primary functions of erythrocytes, leukocytes, and thrombocytes.
6. State the stages of the blood clotting mechanism.

"All the veins and arteries proceed from the heart; and the reason is that the maximum thickness that is found in these veins and arteries is at the junction that they make with the heart; and the farther away they are from the heart the thinner they become and they are divided into more minute ramifications."

—Leonardo da Vinci

KEY TERMS

aorta the largest artery that carries blood from the heart to be distributed by branch arteries through the body

arteriole the small terminal branch of an artery that ends in capillaries

artery a tubular, muscular, and elastic-walled vessel that carries blood from the heart through the body

atria the two chambers of the heart that receive blood from the veins and force it into the ventricles

capillary a small blood vessel connecting arterioles with venules

circulatory system the system that comprises blood, blood vessels, lymphatics, and heart, and is concerned with the circulation of the blood and lymph

coagulation cessation of bleeding; formation of a clot. The clotting process consists of the action of blood vessels, platelets, and coagulation factors.

diastole the resting phase of the heart muscle's contraction

erythrocyte red blood cell

granulocyte a cell with granule-containing cytoplasm

hematopoiesis the formation of blood cells in the body

hemoglobin an iron-containing protein pigment present in red blood cells. It functions primarily to transport oxygen from the lungs to the tissues of the body.

hemostasis the process of coagulation, or clot formation, that repairs vessel damage and stops blood loss

leukocyte white blood cell

lymphocyte a leukocyte produced in the lymphoid tissue

monocyte a large leukocyte formed in bone marrow, with abundant cytoplasm and a kidney-shaped nucleus; ingests bacteria and debris in tissue

pathogens disease-producing agents

peripheral circulation includes both the systemic circulation and the pulmonary circulation

plasma the yellow fluid component of blood

pulmonary circulation the blood flow to the lungs

serum liquid portion of blood without clotting factors

systemic circulation the flow of blood to the body, exclusive of the pulmonary circulation

systole the active, or contracting, phase of the heart muscle's contraction

thrombocyte platelet

tunica adventitia an enclosing tissue that makes up the outer layer of the artery wall

tunica intima the innermost membrane of the artery wall

tunica media the middle layer of the artery wall

vein a vessel that carries blood back to the heart

ventricles the two chambers of the heart that receive blood from the corresponding atria and force it into the arteries

venule a small vein connecting the capillaries with the larger systemic veins

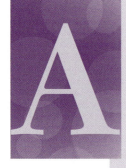

s a member of the clinical laboratory team, the phlebotomist should be familiar with the various tests performed in the laboratory. Tests are designed to assess the functioning status of all of the human body's systems: the integumentary, skeletal, muscular, nervous, sensory, endocrine, circulatory and lymphatic, respiratory, digestive, urinary, and reproductive systems. A sound knowledge of the structure and function of these systems is essential for phlebotomists to understand better why they are collecting a blood sample from a patient. Because the circulatory system is the primary system with which phlebotomists interact in collecting laboratory specimens, this book will discuss that system. Phlebotomists are encouraged to do further reading and to study supplementary materials to expand their knowledge of the other body systems.

The **circulatory system**, or cardiovascular system, is made up of the heart, blood vessels, and blood. The system functions to transport nutrients, waste products, gases, and hormones through the body. In addition, the circulatory system plays an important role in the immune response and the regulation of body temperature.

■ THE HEART

The heart is a muscular pump that forces the blood through the blood vessels. Actually, the heart can be seen as a two-pump system. One pump sends blood to the lungs, and the other pushes blood to all other tissues of the body. The blood flowing to the lungs makes up the **pulmonary circulation**. The blood flowing to the rest of the body makes up the **systemic circulation**. The heart pumps approximately 5 L of blood per minute in a healthy adult. It contracts an average of 70 to 75 times per minute, without stopping, throughout a person's lifetime. The heart is about the size of a closed fist and is located in the thoracic cavity, between the lungs.

The heart consists of four chambers: two **atria** and two **ventricles**. The right atrium receives blood returning from the bodily tissues. This blood is depleted of oxygen and is carried by **veins**. The right ventricle pumps the venous blood received from the right atrium into the lungs. The left atrium receives blood from the lungs that is high in oxygen content. The left ventricle pumps the oxygenated blood back to the bodily tissues. This oxygenated blood travels through arteries. Please refer to Figure 3-1.

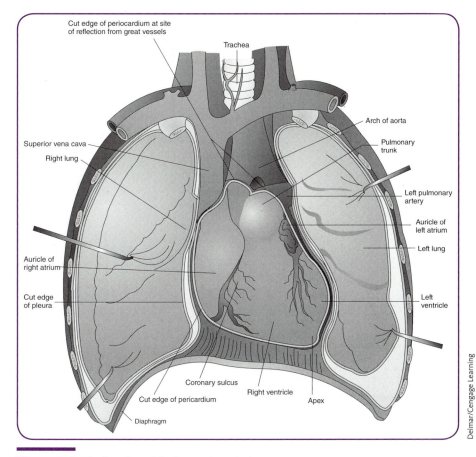

Figure 3-1 caption labels:
Cut edge of periocardium at site of reflection from great vessels
Trachea
Arch of aorta
Pulmonary trunk
Superior vena cava
Left pulmonary artery
Right lung
Auricle of left atrium
Left lung
Auricle of right atrium
Cut edge of pleura
Left ventricle
Coronary sulcus
Right ventricle
Apex
Cut edge of pericardium
Diaphragm

Delmar/Cengage Learning

Figure 3-1 The interior of the heart. *See color insert.*

    The right and left sides of the heart work together. The blood is pushed through the chambers by the heart muscle's contractions. Contractions begin in the atria and are followed by contractions in the ventricles. The active—contracting—phase is called **systole**. It is followed by a resting phase called **diastole**. The atria rest while the ventricles contract. After the ventricles empty, both chambers relax while they fill again with blood. Then the atria contract and the cycle begins again.

■ BLOOD VESSELS

The pulmonary circulation and the systemic circulation together make up the **peripheral circulation**. Please refer to Figure 3-2. The blood vessels and the four heart chambers form a closed system for the flow of

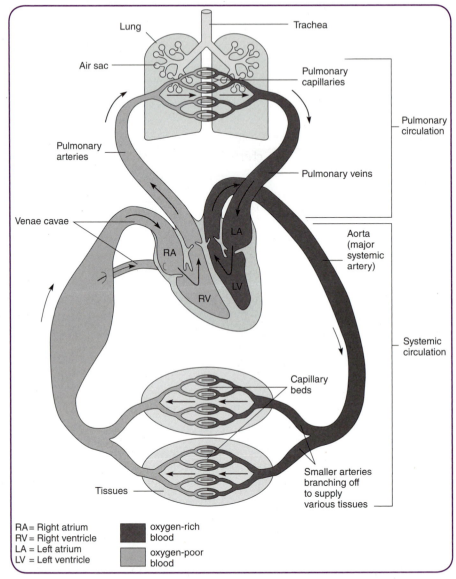

Figure 3-2 Schematic drawing of blood circulation. *See color insert.*

blood. The pulmonary vessels transport blood to and from the lungs. They include the pulmonary artery, capillaries in the lungs, and veins that drain those capillaries. The systemic circulation network consists of the **aorta** and systemic arteries and veins.

Arteries

Arteries are blood vessels that carry blood away from the heart (see Figure 3-3). Blood is pumped from the ventricles into large, elastic arteries. The largest artery is the aorta, about 2.5 centimeters in diameter. It has thick walls because it receives blood under the highest pressure, directly from the left ventricle. The large, elastic arteries branch into smaller arteries. As the arteries grow smaller, they become less elastic and begin to have more smooth (involuntary) muscle tissue. The smallest arteries are called **arterioles**.

Arteries are composed of three layers, or tunics. The innermost membrane, called the **tunica intima**, is a layer of endothelium that forms a smooth surface. This smooth surface enables blood to flow easily through

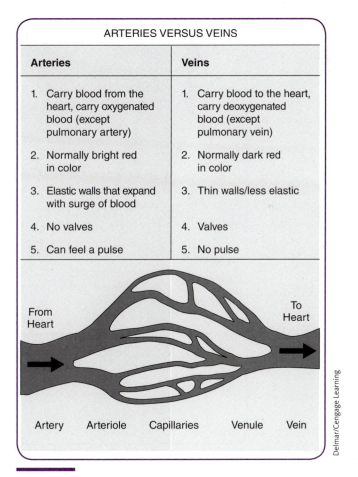

ARTERIES VERSUS VEINS	
Arteries	**Veins**
1. Carry blood from the heart, carry oxygenated blood (except pulmonary artery)	1. Carry blood to the heart, carry deoxygenated blood (except pulmonary vein)
2. Normally bright red in color	2. Normally dark red in color
3. Elastic walls that expand with surge of blood	3. Thin walls/less elastic
4. No valves	4. Valves
5. Can feel a pulse	5. No pulse

From Heart

To Heart

Artery   Arteriole   Capillaries   Venule   Vein

Delmar/Cengage Learning

Figure 3-3 Blood flow from artery to capillary to vein. *See color insert.*

the vessel. The middle layer, or **tunica media**, is the thickest layer and is made of smooth muscle combined with elastic connective tissue. The **tunica adventitia** is the outermost layer, and it is composed of supporting connective tissue. See Figure 3-4.

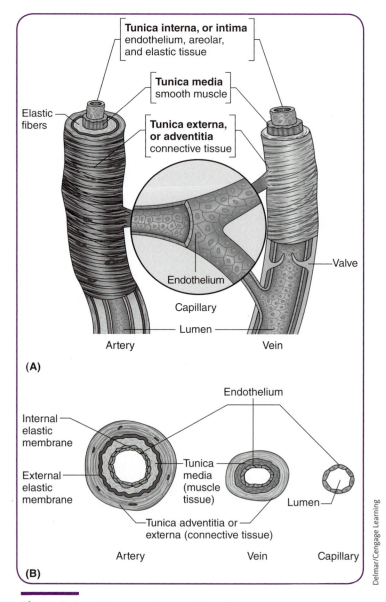

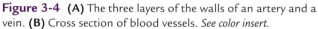

Figure 3-4 (**A**) The three layers of the walls of an artery and a vein. (**B**) Cross section of blood vessels. *See color insert.*

Capillaries

Arterioles transport blood from the small arteries to **capillaries**. There are about 10 billion capillaries in the body. Capillaries are microscopic in size. They are 0.5 to 1 millimeter long, and they branch without a change in their diameter. They have the thinnest walls of all the vessels: a one-cell layer (refer to Figure 3-4). Capillary walls are transparent and consist of endothelium surrounded by a layer of loose connective tissue. Because of the thinness of the walls, direct exchanges between the blood and body cells are made. Red blood cells flow in single file through the capillaries. As the blood flows through the capillaries, it gives up oxygen and nutrients to the tissues. In exchange, it picks up carbon dioxide and other by-products. Blood pressure forces fluid out of the capillaries, and osmosis moves fluid into the capillaries. Blood flow through the capillaries is cyclic, due to the contraction and relaxation of the precapillary sphincters. Precapillary sphincters are smooth muscle cells located at the points where capillaries branch. The contraction and relaxation of the sphincters is regulated by the metabolic needs of the tissues. Blood flow is increased when oxygen levels decrease. Blood flow is also increased when levels of glucose, amino acids, and fatty acids decrease. An increase in carbon dioxide or a decrease in pH (increase in acid level of blood) causes the precapillary sphincters to relax. Please refer to Figure 3-3.

Veins

Blood flows from capillaries into **venules** (see Figure 3-3). Venules are the smallest veins, and their walls are only slightly thicker than those of capillaries. Their diameter is also slightly larger. Venules are composed of endothelium surrounded by a connective-tissue membrane. As the venules connect with small veins, the vessel walls become thicker. Even small veins are larger in diameter than venules. Medium-size veins collect blood from small veins and transport it to large veins. Although their walls become thicker as veins increase in size, veins have much thinner walls than arteries. In addition, the blood they carry is under much lower pressure. Like arteries, veins are composed of three layers, but the veins' middle tunic is thinner.

Veins having diameters greater than 2 millimeters have valves. Valves allow blood to flow toward the heart but not in the opposite direction, and they become more numerous with the increase in the size of the vein. There are more valves in veins of the legs than in veins of the arms. These valves prevent the pull of gravity from drawing the flow of blood down toward the feet.

Phlebotomists come in contact most frequently with the arteries and veins in the upper limbs. Therefore, this discussion of systemic circulation will focus on the upper limbs. The arteries of the upper limbs consist of the following:

- *Subclavian artery,* located just below the clavicle.
- *Brachial artery,* located in the arm; a continuation of the axillary artery.
- *Ulnar artery,* located in the arm; it branches from the brachial to the medial, or little finger, side.
- *Radial artery,* located in the arm; it also branches from the brachial artery, but on the thumb side.

See Figure 3-5 for an overview of the major arteries of the systemic circulation.

The radial artery is the artery used most often in obtaining an arterial blood sample for blood gases (a test ordered to assess lung function by measuring oxygen and other gases of respiration).

The veins of the upper limbs can be divided into two groups:

- The deep veins that run parallel to the arteries. The *brachial veins* are the most noteworthy for our purposes. They accompany the brachial artery and empty into the axillary vein.
- The superficial veins that drain the blood in the arm into the deep veins, including the *cephalic vein,* which empties into the subclavian vein, and the *basilic vein,* which empties into the axillary vein.

See Figure 3-6 for an overview of the major veins of the body.

The phlebotomist will be able to see many of the tributaries of the two major superficial veins through the skin on the patient's forearm and hand. The *median cubital* usually connects the cephalic vein with the basilic vein. The median cubital is usually quite prominent in the cubital fossa, the anterior surface of the upper arm at the elbow, and is an ideal site for performing a venipuncture. Please refer to figure 3-7.

■ BLOOD

Blood is classified as a connective tissue. It is made up of cells and cell fragments moving freely in a liquid substance called **plasma**. Normally the total circulating blood volume is about 8 percent of body weight. About 55 percent of this volume is plasma.

Plasma is a pale yellow fluid consisting of 92 percent water and 8 percent dissolved substances such as proteins, ions, nutrients, gases, waste products, and regulatory substances. Of the cells and cell fragments, or formed elements, in the blood, about 95 percent are red blood cells, or

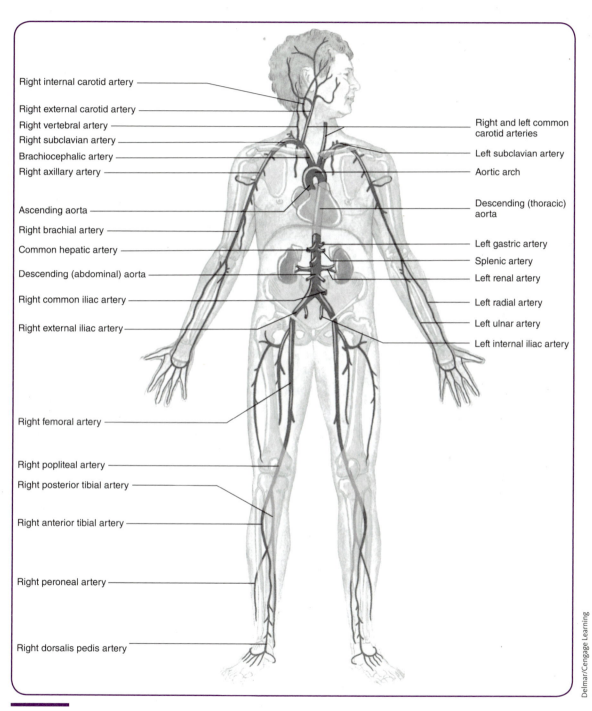

Figure 3-5 The major arteries of the systemic circulation. *See color insert.*

Right internal carotid artery

Right external carotid artery

Right vertebral artery

Right subclavian artery

Brachiocephalic artery

Right axillary artery

Ascending aorta

Right brachial artery

Common hepatic artery

Descending (abdominal) aorta

Right common iliac artery

Right external iliac artery

Right femoral artery

Right popliteal artery

Right posterior tibial artery

Right anterior tibial artery

Right peroneal artery

Right dorsalis pedis artery

Right and left common carotid arteries

Left subclavian artery

Aortic arch

Descending (thoracic) aorta

Left gastric artery

Splenic artery

Left renal artery

Left radial artery

Left ulnar artery

Left internal iliac artery

Delmar/Cengage Learning

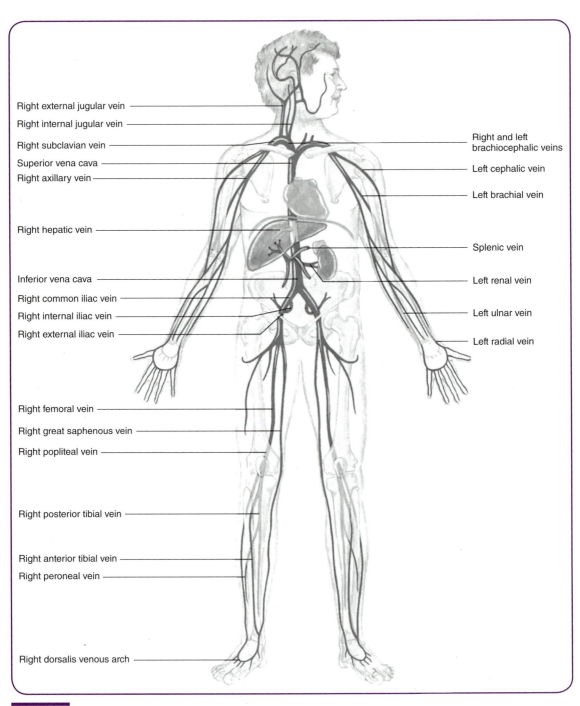

Right external jugular vein

Right internal jugular vein

Right subclavian vein

Superior vena cava

Right axillary vein

Right hepatic vein

Inferior vena cava

Right common iliac vein

Right internal iliac vein

Right external iliac vein

Right femoral vein

Right great saphenous vein

Right popliteal vein

Right posterior tibial vein

Right anterior tibial vein

Right peroneal vein

Right dorsalis venous arch

Right and left
brachiocephalic veins

Left cephalic vein

Left brachial vein

Splenic vein

Left renal vein

Left ulnar vein

Left radial vein

Delmar/Cengage Learning

Figure 3-6 The major veins of the body. *See color insert.*

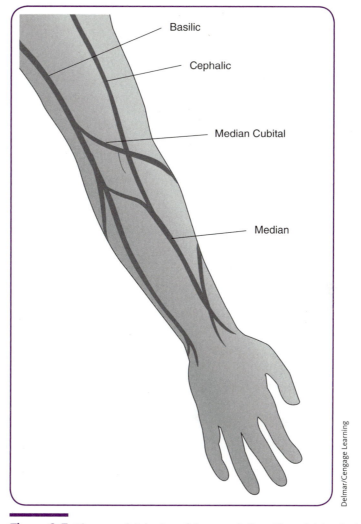

Delmar/Cengage Learning

Figure 3-7 The superficial veins of the arm. *Refer to Figure 5-1 in color insert.*

erythrocytes. Plasma also produces a buffy coat that consists of a layer of yellowish plasma from which the red cells have settled out in coagulated blood. The remaining 5 percent consist of white blood cells, or **leukocytes**, and cell fragments called platelets, or **thrombocytes**. Please refer to Figure 3-8.

The process of blood cell production is called **hematopoiesis**. In the fetus, hematopoiesis occurs in the liver, thymus gland, spleen, lymph

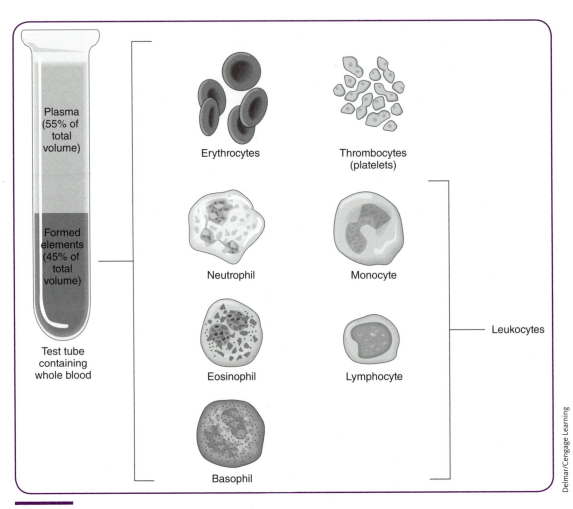

Figure 3-8 The major components of blood. *See color insert.*

nodes, and red bone marrow. In children, red blood cells are produced in the marrow cavities of all the bones, and some white cells are produced in lymphatic tissue. In adults, red blood cells, many white blood cells, and platelets are formed in the bone marrow. By the time an individual reaches age 20, the marrow in the cavities of the long bones, except for the upper humerus and femur, has become inactive. Active marrow is called red marrow, and inactive marrow is called yellow marrow. Yellow marrow is mixed with fat. Bone marrow is one of the largest organs in the body, and is comparable in weight and size to the liver.

Erythrocytes

Erythrocytes, or red blood cells, are manufactured in the bone marrow. They are shaped like concave disks, thinner at the center than at the edges. Erythrocytes live in circulation for about 120 days in men and 110 days in women. The average normal red blood cell count is 5.4 million per cubic microliter of blood in men and 4.8 million per cubic microliter in women. There are approximately 25 trillion red blood cells in a 135-pound man. Approximately 2.5 million red blood cells are produced every second, or 200 million every day. The primary functions of erythrocytes are to carry oxygen from the lungs to various tissues of the body and to assist in the transport of carbon dioxide from the tissues to the lungs. Please refer to Figure 3-9.

Oxygen is transported by **hemoglobin**. Hemoglobin is a pigmented protein that gives blood its red color, and it is responsible for 97 percent of the oxygen transported in blood. Each red blood cell contains approximately 270 million hemoglobin molecules. Iron is necessary for oxygen transport, and approximately two-thirds of the body's iron is found in hemoglobin. About one-third of a red blood cell's volume is hemoglobin.

Leukocytes

Leukocytes, or white blood cells, are another formed element in blood. They are called white blood cells because they are white in color, as they lack hemoglobin. Leukocytes are spherical in shape and are larger than erythrocytes. They have nuclei of varying shapes and sizes. White blood cells normally number 4,000 to 11,000 per microliter of blood. Leukocytes can leave the blood and travel in an amoeba-like fashion through the tissues. They function to protect the body against invading microorganisms, and they remove dead cells and debris from the tissues. Whenever **pathogens** (disease-producing agents) enter the tissues, white blood cells called neutrophils and monocytes proceed by amoeboid movement to the area of infection. Once there, they engulf the pathogens by phagocytosis. Phagocytosis is a process of ingestion and digestion by cells of substances such as bacteria, foreign particles, other cells, and cell debris. If the pathogens are very strong, however, they may destroy the leukocytes. A collection of leukocytes and bacteria forms pus.

There are different types of leukocytes. They are defined by their size, the shape of their nucleus, and the appearance of granules in the cytoplasm. **Granulocytes** are the most numerous of the white blood cells, and they have a horseshoe-shaped nucleus. Granulocytes are divided into *neutrophils, eosinophils,* and *basophils*. The granulocytes have granules

Blood cell		Life span in blood	Function
Erythrocyte	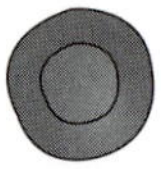	120 days	O_2 and CO_2 transport
Neutrophil	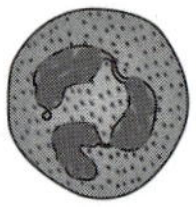	7–12 hours	Immune defenses
Eosinophil	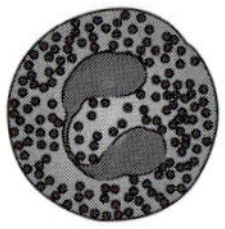	Unknown	Defense against parasites
Basophil	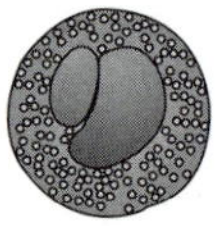	Unknown	Inflammatory response
Monocyte	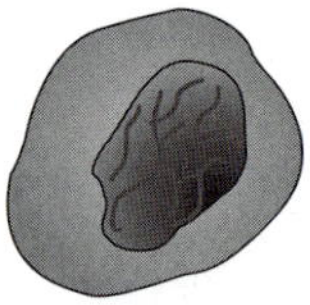	3 days–years	Immune surveillance (precursor of tissue macrophage)
B Lymphocyte	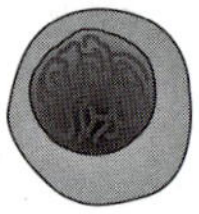	Unknown	Antibody production (precursor of plasma cells)
T Lymphocyte	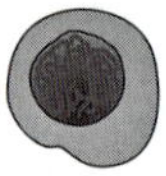	Unknown	Cellular immune response
Platelets	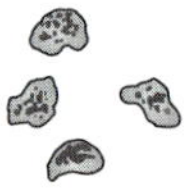	7–8 days	Blood clotting

Delmar/Cengage Learning

Figure 3-9 The function and life span of blood cells. *See color insert.*

that contain active substances involved in inflammatory and allergic reactions. Basophils contain histamine and heparin (heparin also prevents the formation of clots). Eosinophils attack some parasites, and they become active during allergic reactions. The eosinophil level increases in patients with allergic diseases. Eosinophils release chemicals that reduce inflammation. The chemicals also destroy certain worm parasites. Neutrophils seek out, ingest, and kill bacteria. They are the body's first line of defense against bacterial infection. Neutrophils must be reproduced at the rate of 100 billion cells per day to maintain the normal number circulating in the blood. Neutrophils normally live for only 10 to 12 hours. The two other white cell types are **lymphocytes** and **monocytes**. Lymphocytes have large, round nuclei and little cytoplasm. Monocytes have abundant cytoplasm and kidney-shaped nuclei.

The granulocytes, lymphocytes, and monocytes play very specific roles in the body's defense system. Lymphocytes have an important role in the body's immune system. They produce antibodies and other chemicals that destroy pathogens, contribute to allergic reactions, reject grafts, control tumors, and regulate the immune system. Lymphocytes are formed in the bone marrow, lymph nodes, thymus, and spleen. Monocytes enter the blood from the bone marrow and circulate for about 72 hours. They then enter the tissues, where they ingest bacteria, dead neutrophils, cell fragments, and other debris.

The bone marrow and lymph glands continually produce and maintain a reserve of white blood cells. When a pathogen invades the body, reserves are released, and the manufacturing of large quantities of white cells rapidly begins. It is this rapid production of cells that causes fever.

White blood cells react very specifically to different illnesses. Therefore, white cell counts are very important for diagnosing disease. For example, if neutrophils rise from a normal of 60 percent to above 75 percent, pneumonia or appendicitis may be indicated.

Thrombocytes

Thrombocytes, or platelets, are the third formed element in the blood. Platelets are not cells but rather fragments of cells. They are the smallest of the elements in blood. They number 200,000 to 400,000 per cubic microliter of circulating blood, and live for approximately eight days. They are produced in the bone marrow and removed from circulation by the spleen. The megakaryocytes, which are giant cells in the bone marrow, form platelets by pinching off bits of cytoplasm and forcing them into the circulation. About 60 percent to 75 percent of the platelets released from the bone marrow are in the bloodstream, and the remainder are found primarily in the spleen.

Platelets are essential to blood **coagulation**, defined as the formation of a clot. This process is called **hemostasis**. When a small blood vessel is damaged, it initiates a chain of events. First, the smooth muscle in the vessel wall contracts. Contraction of the smooth muscle is directed through neural responses to pain and through chemicals released by platelets. Next, a platelet plug is formed. When a vessel is damaged, the epithelial lining is torn and the connective tissue is exposed. Platelets are activated by the exposed connective tissue; they stick to the tissue and to each other.

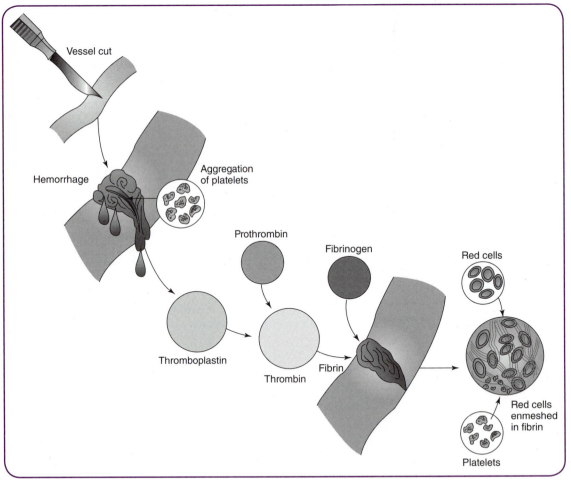

Figure 3-10 The stages of blood clotting. *See color insert.*

The accumulated platelets form a plug that seals the damaged area of the vessel. When platelets are activated, they release several chemicals that decrease blood loss. Serotonin causes blood vessels to constrict, which reduces blood flow. Other chemicals activate additional platelets that attach themselves to the platelet plug. When the vessel damage is severe, platelet plugs are not sufficient to stop the blood flow. Then, instead of a platelet plug, a clot is formed. A clot is a network of protein fibers, called fibrin, that traps blood cells, platelets, and fluid. The clear yellowish liquid that is seen after the clot forms is called **serum**. Serum is blood plasma without the clotting factors. Please refer to Figure 3-10.

[ALERT]

The phlebotomist must use great caution with patients who have prolonged bleeding times. It is important to check the puncture site before leaving the patient to ensure bleeding has stopped. Apply pressure to the site with gauze and bandage appropriately.

SUMMARY

A sound knowledge of the structure and function of the body's systems is essential for the phlebotomist to better understand why a blood sample is being collected from a patient. An understanding of the circulatory system provides the phlebotomist with valuable information while performing venipunctures. Phlebotomists will also better understand blood testing if they know about all systems of the body, including the circulatory system.

REVIEW ACTIVITIES

1. The circulatory system consists of:

   a. _____

   b. _____

   c. _____

2. The active phase of the heart contractions is called _____.

3. The resting phase is called _____.

4. The direction in which arteries carry blood is _____ the heart.

5. The largest artery is the _____.

6. _____ forces fluid out of the capillaries, and moves the fluid into the capillaries.

7. Blood flow _____ when _____ decreases.

8. The arteries of the upper limbs are the:

   a. _____

   b. _____

   c. _____

   d. _____

9. The major superficial veins in the arm are the _____ vein, which empties into the _____ vein, and the _____ vein, which empties into the _____ vein.

10. The median cubital usually connects the _____ vein and the _____ vein.

11. The median cubital is usually quite prominent in the _____.

12. Red blood cells live for _____ days.

13. The pigmented protein that gives blood its red color is called _____.

14. A collection of leukocytes and bacteria forms _____.

15. Leukocytes play an important part in the body's _____.

16. _____ are essential for blood to coagulate.

17. _____ is the yellowish liquid portion of blood.

■ DISCUSSION QUESTIONS

1. Capillary blood flow increases when oxygen levels decrease. What do you think is the reason for this?

2. Discuss the primary functions of erythrocytes, leukocytes, and thrombocytes.

4

Blood Collection Equipment

"Give us the tools, and we will finish the job."

—Winston Churchill

OBJECTIVES

After studying this unit, it is the responsibility of the learner to be able to:

1. Stock a phlebotomy collection tray with the most common blood collection tools and describe the function of each.

2. Demonstrate how a tourniquet is placed on the arm.

3. Explain the different types of needles used for phlebotomy.

4. Describe the different collection tubes and the contents of each tube.

5. Describe the microcollection equipment, including lancets and collection tubes.

anticoagulant any agent that prevents coagulation

Betadine an iodine solution

bevel the slanted edge at the tip of a needle

butterfly needle a needle and tubing connected with a plastic wing-shaped holder that is used for fragile veins; it may be used attached to a syringe or with a luer adapter.

evacuated collection system a venous blood collection system that involves a double-pointed needle and a vacuumized collection tube

gauge needle bore size

gauze loosely woven cotton fabric, available in sterile packets

hub clear, plastic section of a needle

lancet a small surgical blade used to puncture the skin

syringe a device used for drawing out (or injecting) a quantity of fluid

tourniquet a length of rubber or synthetic rubber tied around the arm to arrest blood flow and increase venous filling

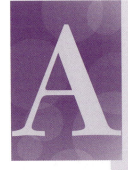ll professionals rely on tools of some type to help them perform a job. Whether it is a carpenter's chisel, a surgeon's scalpel, or a phlebotomist's needle, the tool used must be appropriate for the situation. A carpenter would not use a sledgehammer to drive in a nail when building an oak cabinet. Similarly, a phlebotomist would not use a 21-gauge evacuated-system needle to perform a venipuncture on a fragile hand vein. All professionals must know the tools of their trade.

In today's environment, new and improved products appear on the market continually. However, the standard blood collection tools remain basically unchanged. The phlebotomist's blood collection tools are needles, needle holders, syringes, collection tubes, lancets, tourniquets, skin cleansing agents, **gauze** or cotton balls, tape, gloves, sharps disposal units, and a collection tray, cart, or table for holding supplies. Please refer to Figure 4-1.

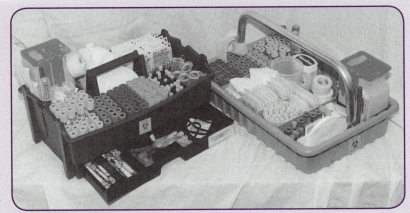

Figure 4-1 Routine venipuncture supplies, part of a phlebotomy collection tray. *See color insert.*

▪ VENIPUNCTURE EQUIPMENT

Cotton Covering

Gauze is a fabric made of loosely woven cotton. Sterile gauze should be kept in its wrapping until ready for use. Do not lay the gauze on any surface other than the inside of the wrapper once the wrapper has been opened. The gauze is applied to the arm immediately upon withdrawal of the needle from the venipuncture site. Apply pressure until the bleeding has stopped. The phlebotomist may fold the gauze pad into quarters and tape it on the puncture site to be used as a pressure bandage.

Cotton balls serve the same purpose as gauze. Cotton is used because it is fibrous and readily takes up fluids. However, cotton balls are not available in sterile packages.

Tourniquet

A **tourniquet** is a pliable strap wrapped around the arm used to temporarily arrest the flow of blood to or from the arm. It increases venous filling, causing the veins to appear more prominent. Because of the problem of latex allergies, it is preferred that disposable non-latex or synthetic rubber tourniquets be used. A tourniquet is approximately 1 inch wide and 18 to 20 inches long. Thicker bands are also available with Velcro attached to the ends. Either type may be used, depending on the phlebotomist's preference. The blood pressure cuff may also be used when veins are difficult to find. A non-disposable tourniquet should be discarded or cleaned immediately if contaminated with blood. It may be cleaned with 70% isopropyl alcohol frequently and disinfected with chlorine bleach dilution of 1:10 if contaminated with blood or other body fluids. In addition, it should have good stretching ability. After multiple uses the tourniquet loses its ability to stretch and should be discarded. At the present time, there are no clear directives or standards concerning the multiple uses of tourniquets. Each health care institution will have its own procedure and policy.

PROCEDURE Applying the Tourniquet

1. Wrap the tourniquet around the arm approximately 3 inches above the bend of the elbow. The tourniquet should be applied 3 to 4 inches above the venipuncture site if the hand or wrist area is to be used. A space of 3 inches allows adequate room for prepping the area and performing the venipuncture without interference from the tourniquet (see Figure 4-2A). A larger space between the site and the tourniquet closes off more of the vein than is necessary.

2. Grasp an end of the tourniquet with each hand so that enough space is left in the middle of the tourniquet to wrap around the

circumference of the patient's arm. Leaving too much or too little space will prevent you from applying the tourniquet with the appropriate amount of tightness.

3. Firmly stretch the tourniquet and bring your hands together.

4. Cross the ends of the tourniquet at the point of your grasp (see Figure 4-2B). Crossing the ends ensures the tightness of the tourniquet. This also allows for easy one-handed release of the tourniquet when it is pulled on one end. The purpose of applying the tourniquet is to increase venous filling, thus making the veins more prominent. A tourniquet that is too loose will not cause venous filling. A tourniquet that is too tight will be uncomfortable for the patient.

5. Approximately 1 inch from the crossing point, tuck a portion of the top length into the bottom length, forming a loop (see Figure 4-2C). Do not tie the tourniquet as if tying a shoe. Both

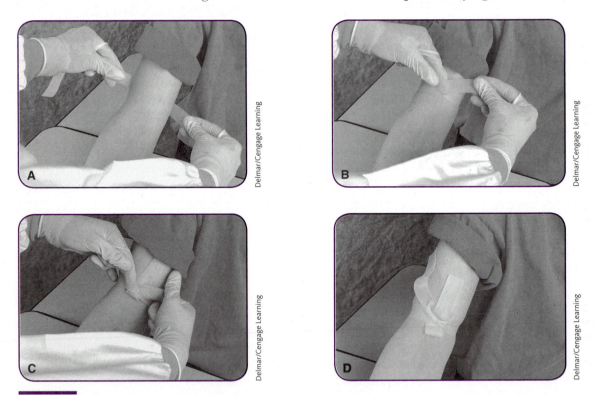

Figure 4-2 Applying a tourniquet. (A) Wrap the tourniquet around the arm approximately 3 inches above the bend of the elbow. (B) Cross the ends of the tourniquet at the point of your grasp. (C) Approximately 1 inch from the crossing point, tuck a portion of the top length into the bottom length, forming a loop. (D) The tourniquet should be snug, but not so tight that the patient's skin is pinched.

ends of the tourniquet should be clear of the puncture site. The tourniquet should be snug, but not so tight that the patient's skin is pinched (see Figure 4-2D).

6. Have the patient make a fist and hyperextend the arm. Do not instruct the patient to "pump" the fist. Pumping the fist may alter some test result values. Notice how the veins become more prominent.

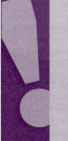

[ALERT]

The tourniquet should not be left on the patient's arm for longer than 1 minute. Leaving it on longer not only causes discomfort to the patient but can affect the results of some laboratory tests.

Disinfectant

Alcohol preps are sterile pads saturated with 70 percent isopropyl alcohol. Alcohol prep pads are used to disinfect the patient's skin before puncturing. Other disinfectants used to cleanse the arm thoroughly include **Betadine** pads and swabs, which contain iodine, a more powerful cleanser for the venipuncture area.

Needles

A variety of needle types and sizes are available to the phlebotomist. Each health care facility supplies its phlebotomists with the brands preferred by its particular laboratory. The needle is composed of the **hub** or plastic section, the shaft, and the **bevel**, or slanted tip. Please refer to Figure 4-3.

Needles vary in length and diameter. The phlebotomist will select the appropriate size needle for each venipuncture, based on the physical characteristics of the patient's vein and the volume of blood required for the ordered test(s). The length of the needle may vary from 1 to 2 inches. Many phlebotomists prefer the 1-inch needle, because it gives them more of a feeling of "control" when they rest their fourth and fifth fingers on the patient's arm for stability. The bore size, or **gauge**, of the needle also varies. The phlebotomist may use 19-gauge to 23-gauge needles (the larger

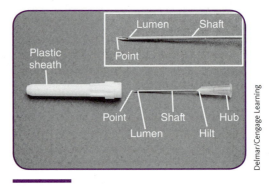

Figure 4-3 Parts of a needle.

the number, the smaller the bore). A small vein requires a small-gauge needle, for instance a 23-gauge. The blood will flow more slowly because of the small diameter of the needle, but the vein will be less likely to collapse. A normal-size vein would require a 20-gauge or 21-gauge needle. Blood donors require a larger sized needle, for instance a 16-gauge needle.

There are generally three types of needles used by the phlebotomist: the multiple-sample needle used as part of the **evacuated collection system** (a system that uses a double-pointed needle and collection tubes that contain a vacuum), the hypodermic needle used with syringes, and the wing-tipped (butterfly) needle.

Multiple-Sample Needle

The most common and most preferred method for venous blood collection is the evacuated system. It is the most efficient and the safest collection method for the phlebotomist. The needle (please refer to Figure 4-4A) has two sharp ends: one end designed to perform the venipuncture and the other to penetrate the rubber stopper of the collection tube. The end penetrating the stopper is shorter in length and is covered with a rubber sleeve. This end is to be screwed into a needle holder (also called a barrel or an adapter). This is a plastic device designed to hold the needle and the collection tube. The rubber sleeve on the needle prevents blood from leaking from the needle as each collection tube is removed from the holder.

One type of multiple-sample needle Punctur-Guard by BioPlexus utilizes an internal blunt safety technology. The needle has a device that allows it to be blunted prior to removal from the patient's vein. Because the needle is blunt when removed from the vein, the potential for an accidental needlestick is eliminated. The needle may be blunted immediately after puncturing the vein, and allows for several vacuum tubes to be collected while blunted. It is particularly effective in drawing a combative patient. However, the needle cannot be repositioned should the blood flow be lost. The SafetyGlide blood collection system by Becton Dickinson utilizes a safety shield covering the needle. The movable shield is pushed along the cannula with the thumb to enclose the needle tip after venipuncture. Sims Portex Needle Pro holder also comes with an attached holder. Please refer to Figure 4-4B.

Hypodermic Needle

The hypodermic needle is attached to a syringe. Needle sizes for venipuncture are 22-gauge, 21-gauge, and 20-gauge. Syringes are required to have a safety shield to cover the needle immediately after use.

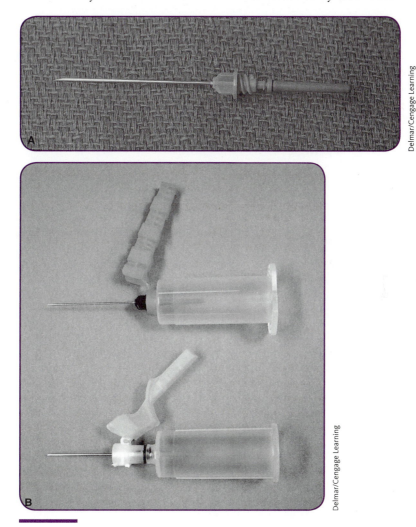

Figure 4-4 (A) Evacuated blood collection system needle. (B) Evacuated blood collection system needles holder. Sims Portex Needle Pro holder (top). Becton Dickinson Eclipse Needle (bottom).

Wing-Tipped (Butterfly) Needle

The **butterfly needle** consists of a needle attached to tubing with a connector on the end. The connector attaches to a syringe or a needle holder. The needle gets its name from the plastic "wings" placed between the needle and the tubing, which is used as a holder for the needle. A plastic safety cover is moved forward over the needle when it is removed from the vein. The phlebotomist may use this needle on fragile veins when only a small volume of blood needs to be drawn. (Please refer to Figure 4-5.)

Needle Holder

The purpose of the needle holder is to hold the needle in place while it penetrates the rubber stopper of the vacuum tube. The holder is made of plastic, and has a variety of safety functions depending upon the manufacturer. One holder has a hinged cover that recaps the needle. Another holder allows the needle to be retracted into the holder. All needle holders are for one-time use only, and should be discarded immediately after use.

Syringe

A **syringe** (please refer to Figure 4-6) is used with the hypodermic or the butterfly needle. Syringes may be used as an alternative method to

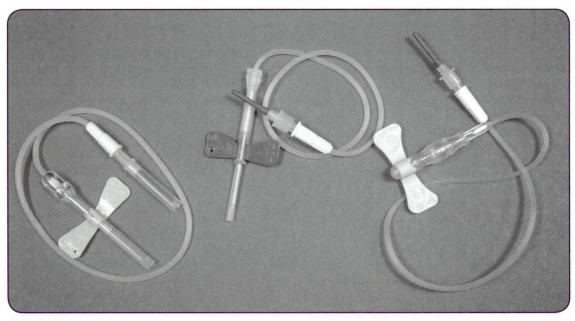

Delmar/Cengage Learning

Figure 4-5 Butterfly collection set.

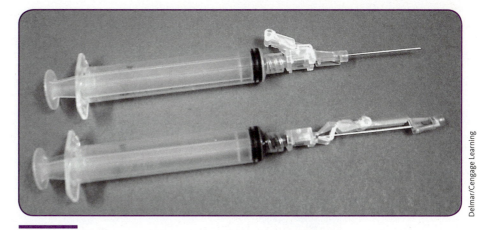

Delmar/Cengage Learning

Figure 4-6 Syringe.

the evacuated system for venous collection when veins are small or fragile. Syringes are most frequently made of plastic. The syringe consists of a barrel and a plunger. It is manufactured with the plunger inside of the barrel. The plunger must be pulled back slowly to withdraw blood from the vein. Often when the syringe is manufactured, the plunger will stick inside of the barrel. When assembling your equipment, you should pull back on the plunger to approximately two inches and then push the plunger back to the original position. Repeat the procedure two to three times. This will allow the plunger to move smoothly when pulling blood into the syringe. Syringes come in a variety of sizes. The barrel of the syringe is graduated into milliliters. Syringes are normally used when performing a venipuncture on small veins or when the patient's vein presents the possibility of collapsing when using the evacuated system.

Blood Transfer Device

A blood transfer device is a plastic holder that is utilized to transfer blood safely from the syringe into a blood collection tube. Becton Dickinson manufactures a holder with a pre-attached multiple sample female luer adapter. The syringe containing a blood sample is locked into one end of the holder and a collection tube is inserted and pushed into the opposite end of the holder, allowing the luer adapter to puncture the rubber stopper of the tube. A needle on the syringe is not necessary to perform the transfer. The vacuum in the collection tube will allow the tube to fill with blood. Please refer to Figure 4-7.

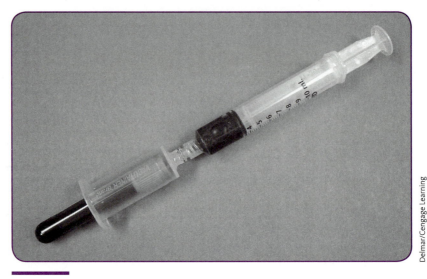

Delmar/Cengage Learning

Figure 4-7 Blood transfer device. *See color insert.*

Blood Collection Tubes

The evacuated system uses vacuumized collection tubes made of plastic or glass. The tubes vary in size and have color-coded rubber stoppers that indicate the type of additive in the tube. Please refer to Figure 4-8 and Table 4-1. Additives include:

- **Anticoagulants** that prevent coagulation, or the clotting of blood. One purpose of anticoagulants is to extend the metabolism and life of the red blood cells after collection. Another purpose is to provide plasma for certain tests. The anticoagulants used include oxalate, citrate, heparin, and ethylenediaminetetracetate (EDTA). Citrates, oxalate, and EDTA remove calcium and form insoluble calcium salts that prevent coagulation. EDTA prevents platelet aggregation and is used for platelet counts and platelet function tests. EDTA also allows for minimal distortion of white blood cells when preparing blood films. Heparin inactivates thrombin and thromboplastin, which are blood-clotting chemicals. The correct ratio of blood to anticoagulant is very important. An incorrect amount of anticoagulant may cause inaccurate test results.

- **Separating gel**, which forms a barrier between the plasma or serum and the cells.

- **Clot activators**, which decrease the clotting time of blood.

BD Vacutainer® Venous Blood Collection

Tube Guide

For the full array of BD Vacutainer® Blood Collection Tubes, visit www.bd.com/vacutainer.
Many are available in a variety of sizes and draw volumes (for pediatric applications). Refer to our website for full descriptions.

BD Vacutainer® Tubes with BD Hemogard™ Closure	BD Vacutainer® Tubes with Conventional Stopper	Additive	Inversions at Blood Collection*	Laboratory Use	Your Lab's Draw Volume/Remarks
Gold	Red/ Gray	• Clot activator and gel for serum separation	5	For serum determinations in chemistry. May be used for routine blood donor screening and diagnostic testing of serum for infectious disease.** Tube inversions ensure mixing of clot activator with blood. Blood clotting time: 30 minutes.	
Light Green	Green/ Gray	• Lithium heparin and gel for plasma separation	8	For plasma determinations in chemistry. Tube inversions ensure mixing of anticoagulant (heparin) with blood to prevent clotting.	
Red	Red	• Silicone coated (glass) • Clot activator, Silicone coated (plastic)	0 5	For serum determinations in chemistry. May be used for routine blood donor screening and diagnostic testing of serum for infectious disease.** Tube inversions ensure mixing of clot activator with blood. Blood clotting time: 60 minutes.	
Orange	Gray/ Yellow	• Thrombin	8	For stat serum determinations in chemistry. Tube inversions ensure mixing of clot activator (thrombin) to activate clotting.	
Royal Blue		• Clot activator (plastic serum) • K₂EDTA (plastic)	8 8	For trace-element, toxicology, and nutritional-chemistry determinations. Special stopper formulation provides low levels of trace elements (see package insert). Tube inversions ensure mixing of either clot activator or anticoagulant (EDTA) with blood.	
Green	Green	• Sodium heparin • Lithium heparin	8 8	For plasma determinations in chemistry. Tube inversions ensure mixing of anticoagulant (heparin) with blood to prevent clotting.	
Gray	Gray	• Potassium oxalate/ sodium fluoride • Sodium fluoride/Na₂ EDTA • Sodium fluoride (serum tube)	8 8 8	For glucose determinations. Oxalate and EDTA anticoagulants will give plasma samples. Sodium fluoride is the antiglycolytic agent. Tube inversions ensure proper mixing of additive with blood.	
Tan		• K₂EDTA (plastic)	8	For lead determinations. This tube is certified to contain less than .01 µg/mL(ppm) lead. Tube inversions prevent clotting.	
	Yellow	• Sodium polyanethol sulfonate (SPS) • Acid citrate dextrose additives (ACD): Solution A - 22.0 g/L trisodium citrate, 8.0 g/L citric acid, 24.5 g/L dextrose Solution B - 13.2 g/L trisodium citrate, 4.8 g/L citric acid, 14.7 g/L dextrose	8 8 8	SPS for blood culture specimen collections in microbiology. ACD for use in blood bank studies, HLA phenotyping, and DNA and paternity testing. Tube inversions ensure mixing of anticoagulant with blood to prevent clotting.	
Lavender	Lavender	• Liquid K₃EDTA (glass) • Spray-coated K₂EDTA (plastic)	8 8	K₂EDTA and K₃EDTA for whole blood hematology determinations. K₂EDTA may be used for routine immunohematology testing, and blood donor screening.*** Tube inversions ensure mixing of anticoagulant (EDTA) with blood to prevent clotting.	
White		• K₂EDTA with gel	8	For use in molecular diagnostic test methods (such as, but not limited to, polymerase chain reaction [PCR] and/or branched DNA [bDNA] amplification techniques.) Tube inversions ensure mixing of anticoagulant (EDTA) with blood to prevent clotting.	
Pink	Pink	• Spray-coated K₂EDTA (plastic)	8	For whole blood hematology determinations. May be used for routine immunohematology testing and blood donor screening.*** Designed with special cross-match label for patient information required by the AABB. Tube inversions prevent clotting.	
Light Blue	Light Blue	• Buffered sodium citrate 0.105 M (≈3.2%) glass 0.109 M (3.2%) plastic • Citrate, theophylline, adenosine, dipyridamole (CTAD)	3-4 3-4	For coagulation determinations. CTAD for selected platelet function assays and routine coagulation determination. Tube inversions ensure mixing of anticoagulant (citrate) to prevent clotting.	
Clear					
Clear	New Red/ Light Gray	• None (plastic)	0	For use as a discard tube or secondary specimen tube.	

Note: BD Vacutainer® Tubes for pediatric and partial draw applications can be found on our website.

BD Diagnostics
Preanalytical Systems
1 Becton Drive
Franklin Lakes, NJ 07417 USA

BD Global Technical Services: 1.800.631.0174
vacutainer_techservices@bd.com
BD Customer Service: 1.888.237.2762
www.bd.com/vacutainer

* Invert gently, do not shake
** The performance characteristics of these tubes have not been established for infectious disease testing in general; therefore, users must validate the use of these tubes for their specific assay-instrument/reagent system combinations and specimen storage conditions.
*** The performance characteristics of these tubes have not been established for immunohematology testing in general; therefore, users must validate the use of these tubes for their specific assay-instrument/reagent system combinations and specimen storage conditions.

BD, BD Logo and all other trademarks are property of Becton, Dickinson and Company. © 2008 BD

Printed in USA   08/08   VS5229-9

Figure 4-8 Evacuated collection tube guide. *See color insert.*

VACUUM COLLECTION TUBES

Additive Group	Color Top	General Use	Specimen Type
Polymer gel/silica activator	Gold	Chemistry	Serum
Polymer gel/silica activator	Red/Gray	Chemistry	Serum
None	Red	Chemistry/ Blood Bank	Serum
Sodium Heparin	Green	Chemistry	Plasma
Ammonium Heparin	Green	Chemistry	Plasma
Lithium Heparin	Green	Chemistry	Plasma
Potassium Oxalate, Sodium Fluoride	Lt. Gray	Chemistry	Plasma
K3 EDTA 15% Solution	Lavender	Chemistry	Whole Blood
K3 EDTA 7.5% Solution	Lavender	Hematology	Whole Blood
Citric Acid	Blue	Coagulation	Plasma
2.1 mg Citric Acid	Lt. Blue	Coagulation	Plasma
1.5 ml ACD Solution A	Yellow	Blood Bank	Whole Blood
EDTA	Pink	Blood Bank	Whole Blood
Sodium Heparin	Royal Blue	Toxicology	Plasma

TABLE 4-1 Vacuum Collection Tubes

Delmar/Cengage Learning

Disposal Units

Sharps disposal units come in a variety of shapes and sizes. They are made of a nonpenetrable plastic. The needle holder and the needle must be disposed of in one movement per OSHA. Please refer to Figure 4-9.

Tape

A variety of tapes and bandages are available. Paper tape is excellent for use on delicate skin, especially for elderly patients.

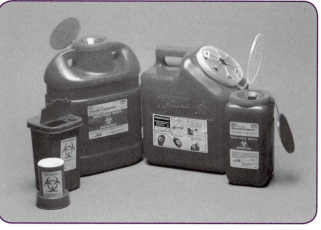

Delmar/Cengage Learning

Figure 4-9 Puncture-proof sharps containers. *See color insert.*

Gloves

Gloves come in a variety of sizes and styles. They are made of latex and non-latex and are usually not sterile. Some gloves do come with powder inside to minimize perspiration inside the gloves, but when specimen processing is involved, the powder is a potential contaminant. Powder-free gloves are recommended for phlebotomists. The phlebotomist should take the time to find a glove size that fits snugly but is not too tight.

■ CAPILLARY PUNCTURE EQUIPMENT

Lancet

A blood **lancet** may be metal or plastic with a metal tip. Lancets come in different point sizes for fingersticks and heelsticks. Their predetermined puncture sizes prevent uncontrolled penetration. Lancets are manufactured in different sizes to provide the appropriate depth of puncture. A range of appropriate depths is utilized for premature babies up to adults. Spring-loaded puncture devices allow for very quick punctures. These devices have a blade-retraction mechanism that is safer for the phlebotomist to use. They come with finger platforms and end caps that must be disposed of after each use. Please refer to Figure 4-10.

Blood-Collecting Devices

Capillary blood collection devices come in many different forms. Your health care facility will decide which types are preferred. Capillary pipettes, microtubes, and the Unopette system for collecting diluted specimens for

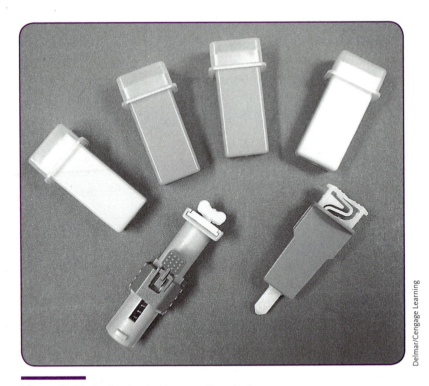

Delmar/Cengage Learning

Figure 4-10 Spring-loaded lancets. *See color insert.*

blood cell counts are among the devices used for capillary blood collection. Please refer to Figure 4-11 and Figure 4-12.

Phlebotomy Collection Tray

A phlebotomy collection tray is utilized to hold specimen collection equipment. The tray is transported by the phlebotomist to the patient's beside, and should be well stocked continuously throughout the day. Outpatient collection sites normally do not utilize collection trays and use a table with drawers to hold collection supplies. Collection trays come in a variety of shapes, sizes, and colors. Stocked carts may also be used as a means for transporting specimen collection supplies. The health care facility will determine the appropriate tray, cart, or table for its specialized purposes. All trays, tables, and carts should be appropriately sanitized on a regular basis. Please refer to Figure 4-1.

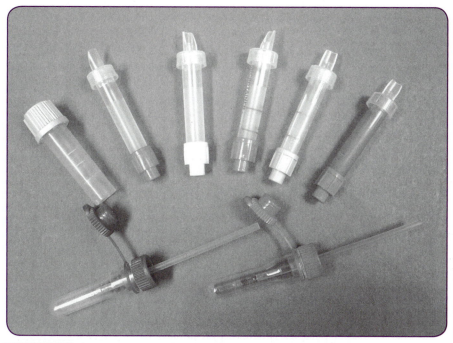

Figure 4-11 Microcollection tubes. *See color insert.*

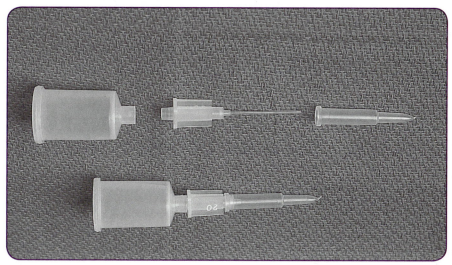

Figure 4-12 Unopette blood diluting unit. *See color insert.*

■ SUMMARY

One of the most important tasks for the phlebotomist is to learn how to use blood-drawing equipment properly. Experience will help the phlebotomist to choose the right equipment for each patient's unique situation. Phlebotomists will continually be exposed to refined equipment that can be utilized to get the best specimen with the least amount of trouble for the patient.

■ REVIEW ACTIVITIES

1. Gauze is made of _____
   _____.

2. Gauze should be placed on the _____ rather than on another surface when preparing to perform a venipuncture, in order to _____
   _____.

3. A tourniquet is used to _____
   _____.

4. A tourniquet should be cleaned and decontaminated frequently because _____
   _____.

5. Alcohol preps are used to _____
   _____.

6. The size of the needle for a venipuncture is chosen based on
   _____
   _____.

7. The three types of needles used most often by the phlebotomist are:

   a. _____

   b. _____

   c. _____

8. The two parts of a syringe are:

   a. _____

   b. _____

9. Identify the additive in the following color-coded collection tubes:

   a. Lavender _____

   b. Blue _____

   c. Green _____

   d. Red-brown _____

   e. Gray _____

   f. Pink _____

   g. Yellow _____

■ DISCUSSION QUESTION

1. You go to Room 606 to draw the patient in bed 1. You also have lab orders to draw the patient in bed 2. The patient in bed 1 is an 80-year-old male with very small, fragile veins. The patient in bed 2 is a 20-year-old male with large, healthy veins. Why is it important to know the function and qualities of the equipment in your collection tray?

5 Collection by Routine Venipuncture

OBJECTIVES

After studying this unit, it is the responsibility of the learner to be able to:

1. Organize a workload by stat, timed, ASAP, and routine orders.
2. Explain the importance of accurately identifying the patient.
3. Write the process for patient identification for outpatients and inpatients.
4. Describe the process taken should the patient not have an inpatient or outpatient identification armband.
5. Demonstrate the positioning of the patient for venipuncture.
6. Demonstrate and explain the process of venipuncture site selection.
7. Demonstrate appropriate venipuncture technique on an injectable training arm.
8. Demonstrate appropriate venipuncture technique on a fellow student.
9. List the appropriate order of draw when using the evacuated collection system.
10. List the rationale for each step of the venipuncture procedure.
11. Demonstrate on an injectable training arm the appropriate steps in performing a venipuncture with the butterfly winged infusion set.
12. List the appropriate order of draw when using the syringe/butterfly collection.
13. Explain the rationale for using a butterfly/syringe rather than the evacuated collection system.

"Our highly sophisticated and well-controlled laboratory technology is useless if the specimens presented for analysis are already riddled with error because of faulty identification or poor collection techniques. Proper specimen collection and specimen handling are of the utmost importance, for today, errors are more likely to occur in these areas than during the laboratory procedure itself."

—National Committee for Clinical Laboratory Standards (1989)

antecubital in front of the elbow

ASAP as soon as possible

aseptic free from infection

basilic vein prominent vein of the forearm located on the inside edge of the antecubital fossa

cephalic vein prominent vein in the forearm utilized for venipuncture

edematous swollen due to an accumulation of excess fluid in the tissue

hematoma a swelling or mass of blood, usually clotted, in an organ or tissue, caused by a ruptured blood vessel due to injury

hemoconcentration increased localized blood concentration of molecules such as cells, proteins, and coagulation factors

lymphostasis lack of fluid drainage in the lymph system; stoppage of lymph flow

median cubital vein vein in the antecubital area that is most commonly used for venipuncture

routine collection orders collected per individual laboratory policy

stat at once, immediately; from the Latin *statim*

thrombosed occluded, or blocked, by a blood clot

timed collection orders collected at a specified collection time

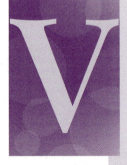enipuncture is the most frequently used method for obtaining a blood sample for diagnostic testing. Because test results are highly dependent on the quality of the specimen, the phlebotomist must perform the venipuncture procedure at a high level of skill. In addition to providing the laboratory with high-quality blood specimens, the phlebotomist must also deliver a high-quality venipuncture to the patient. The procedure must be performed so as to cause minimal trauma to the patient.

This chapter will cover the procedure involved in collecting a blood sample by performing a routine venipuncture. A routine venipuncture assumes that the blood will be drawn from one of the three prominent veins in the **antecubital** area which is in front of the elbow; the median, the **median cubital**, and the median **cephalic** veins. The veins will be punctured using the evacuated collection system or the syringe/butterfly collection system. Because venipuncture is an invasive procedure, it must be performed in an **aseptic** manner, free from the possibility of infection.

The phlebotomist must collect high-quality blood samples and demonstrate expertise in venipuncture technique at all times. Because the student will experience a learning curve, the first several venipunctures may be unsuccessful. The venipuncture may not produce a blood sample, the needle may come out of the puncture prematurely, or a **hematoma** may be produced. These complicating factors will be addressed at the conclusion of the chapter.

While classroom instruction is necessary, it is empirical, or hands-on, experience that will provide the phlebotomist with the opportunity to become proficient in performing blood collections by venipuncture. Venipuncture is a skill, and it must be practiced.

The phlebotomy student should perform all initial venipunctures under the guidance of an instructor. An injectable training arm is an excellent tool to use when attempting the first few venipunctures. It allows the phlebotomist to practice tying the tourniquet, to become familiar with handling the equipment, and to commit to memory the steps in the collection process. Once phlebotomy students feel comfortable with the injectable arm, they may progress to practicing on a fellow student or an instructor. After an appropriate skill level is reached, the phlebotomy student may have the opportunity to obtain blood from a patient under an instructor's guidance.

As previously mentioned, it is very important that the patient receive a venipuncture that is performed in an efficient, aseptic, and relatively painless manner. The preliminary steps to performing the puncture are important and must be carried out in a consistent manner.

■ ORGANIZATION OF WORKLOAD

Prioritize Orders

Collection orders are usually prioritized according to *stat, timed, ASAP,* and *routine* orders. Should the phlebotomist have multiple collections to perform, the orders must be placed in the proper order of collection. **Stat**, or urgent, orders are to be collected immediately and the specimens delivered to the lab immediately. Stat orders have priority in collection over all other orders. They will always be drawn first. **Timed collection** orders must be collected as close to the specified collection time as possible. After stats, timed collections are ranked next in priority. Orders designated **ASAP** (as soon as possible) should be given third priority. **Routine collections** receive last priority, and should be collected per individual laboratory policy.

Review the Collection Requisition

Before greeting a patient or entering a patient's room, review the collection order for the name of the patient, the test(s) ordered, the collection priority, and additional collection instructions or comments. Being prepared beforehand will establish an atmosphere of confidence. Check the collection tray or your work area beforehand as well as the patient's room to make sure the appropriate equipment is available. Be sure to check for special comments on the collection order or for posted instructions in the patient's room. Being alert to special considerations concerning the patient's condition (for example, the patient who may be blind, deaf, or unable to speak English) will help you to be more sensitive to the patient's needs. It will also allow you to appear more professional and well prepared.

■ INTERACTING WITH THE PATIENT

Greet the Patient

Address the patient with a pleasant tone of voice and a smile. Introduce yourself by first name. In a hospital setting, state your purpose in being in the patient's room. If the patient is sleeping, attempt to wake the patient up before you continue with the collection process. The patient may ask questions concerning the tests that have been ordered. Instruct the patient to direct such questions to the physician. If the patient should be unconscious, always address the patient using the same manner and protocol as if he were awake.

Identify the Patient

Absolute identification of the patient is mandatory for every collection. You must ensure accurate identification of the patient and the blood samples throughout the collection process. Failure to do so may result in serious consequences for the patient.

Inpatients

Compare the patient's identification bracelet with the collection order form. Compare the patient's name, identification number, and date of birth. The identification bracelet must be attached to the patient's body. A bracelet taped to the bed is not sufficient. Report any discrepancies or any patients without bracelets to the appropriate person. Do not collect any blood samples until the patient has been absolutely identified.

Outpatients

Ask the patient to state his or her name and birth date. Compare the stated information with the collection order form. Report any discrepancies to the appropriate person. Do not collect a blood sample until discrepancies have been corrected. Some health care facilities issue the patient a temporary identification armband. Verify that the armband contains correct information.

Unidentified Emergency Patients

A temporary means of identifying the patient must be established. The temporary identification must be attached to the patient's body. Do not collect any blood samples until some identification has been attached to the patient.

Verify Diet Restrictions and Time Requirements

Some tests have requirements, such as fasting or a special diet prior to collection of a blood sample. A timed collection should be collected at the specified time. Should any of the diet or time requirements be neglected, accurate test results will not be ensured. Do not collect a blood sample if such requirements have not been met. Report discrepancies to the appropriate person. Should a decision by the appropriate person be made to collect a specimen even though the specimen requirements have not been met, collect the sample and document the discrepancy in the appropriate manner.

Position the Patient

The patient should be positioned so as to be comfortable before the venipuncture is performed. In addition, the patient must be positioned to facilitate comfortable collection for the phlebotomist.

Inpatients

Raise or lower the patient's bed so that it will be at a comfortable level for you when performing the venipuncture. The bed should be at a level that will not create a strain on your back. Have the patient lie on his or her back in a comfortable position. Ask the patient to hyperextend the arm in a straight line from shoulder to wrist. The hand should be lower than the shoulder. A pillow placed under the elbow makes a nice support for the arm. Lower the bed railing only on the side of the bed where you will need to stand. Do not remove any patient restraints. Should the patient be comatose or unable to change position, ask for assistance from the patient's nurse. Do not place the collection tray on the patient's bed; the patient may inadvertently knock the tray off the bed.

Outpatients

The patient should be seated in the drawing chair. Have the patient extend the arm to form a straight line from the shoulder to the wrist. The arm should not be bent at the elbow. The arm rest attached to the drawing chair should support the patient's arm. Most drawing stations have a bed where a blood draw can be performed. Use this bed if you think the patient might faint.

Reassure the Patient

Explain the procedure to the patient. Explain that the pain will be brief. Instruct the patient to remain as relaxed and calm as possible. If the patient appears to be frightened and anxious, have him or her focus on breathing slowly and deeply.

■ PREPARING FOR THE VENIPUNCTURE

Select the Venipuncture Site

By making a preliminary assessment of the best veins in the patient's arms, you will be able to determine the most appropriate equipment for performing the venipuncture. An assessment of the veins will determine whether an evacuated system or a syringe setup will be more appropriate. In addition, you will be able to determine needle size. A preliminary assessment will also identify any need to preheat the puncture site if the blood vessels require dilating. The most frequently used veins for venipuncture are the superficial veins located in the forearm and hand. Please refer to Figure 5-1.

The larger median cubital and cephalic veins are used most often. An alternative choice may be the **basilic vein.** Beginning students should take great care in selecting the basilic vein for venipuncture, as the vein lies in close proximity to the median nerve and the brachial artery. Accidentally nicking the nerve or the artery may cause serious consequences for the patient. However, other veins in the anterior surface of the forearm, as well as in the wrist and hand, are acceptable sites for venipuncture, provided that the selected site has no scarring, hematoma, burn, or edema. The veins on the palm side of the wrist should not be used. Tendons and nerves lie close to the veins, and may be accidentally injured while performing a venipuncture. The venipuncture site should also preferably not be on the side of a mastectomy or on the arm receiving intravenous therapy. There are, however, precautions that may be taken if it is necessary to obtain a blood specimen from a site in either of these two cases. These special considerations will be discussed later in this chapter. If the potential venipuncture site involves any of these conditions, you must try to select a different site.

The phlebotomist should depend primarily on touch and not sight in locating and selecting a vein for venipuncture. A healthy vein will feel "bouncy" to the touch when it is palpated. A **thrombosed** vein, which will not provide an adequate blood sample, feels cordlike and has no spring or bounce. Applying a tourniquet and closing the patient's hand into a fist will cause the veins to fill and become more prominent. Do not pump the fist. Opening and closing the fist rapidly can cause localized **hemoconcentration**, resulting in inaccurate test results.

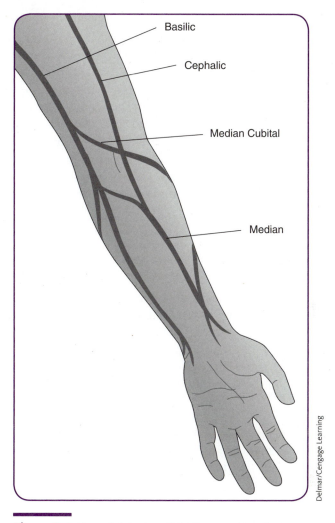

Basilic

Cephalic

Median Cubital

Median

Delmar/Cengage Learning

Figure 5-1 Superficial veins of the forearm. *See color insert.*

Feel, Roll, Trace, Palpate

Feel the vein with your index finger. *Roll* your finger back and forth over the vein to determine its size. *Trace* the vein to determine its path. *Palpate* the vein to determine its resiliency. While selecting a venipuncture site, do not leave the tourniquet on the patient's arm for more than 1 minute. Leaving a tourniquet on longer may cause erroneous results in some lab tests, as well as discomfort for the patient. Look for the best possible vein that will provide an adequate blood sample. The *first vein* to assess would be the *median cubital,* followed by the cephalic vein. If neither vein is adequate, check other superficial forearm, wrist, and hand veins. If you should have difficulty locating a vein, apply hot, moist towels around the venipuncture site (some facilities provide a packaged heating product that is easier to use). Heat will cause the veins to dilate. If you still have problems in palpating the vein, a blood pressure cuff may be used as a tourniquet. Inflate it to approximately 100 mm Hg. You will need to practice this procedure before attempting it on a patient. Deflate the cuff immediately after locating an appropriate vein. If you wish to use the cuff instead of a tourniquet while performing the venipuncture, deflate the cuff to 40 to 50 mm Hg after dilating the vein.

Complicating Factors

There are several factors that can complicate the selection of a venipuncture site:

- *Intravenous therapy* Blood samples should not be drawn from an arm that is receiving an intravenous infusion. Collect blood samples from the patient's other arm. Blood drawn above the intravenous site will be diluted with the fluid being administered, and will cause erroneous test results. If intravenous lines are running in both arms, or if other factors make it impossible to draw a specimen from the other arm, you have some options. One would be to ask the patient's nurse to turn off the intravenous line for a minimum of two minutes. Another would be to apply the tourniquet below the intravenous site. Select a vein other than the one with the intravenous line. You can also withdraw 5 mL of blood and discard it before drawing the test specimens. If coagulation tests are ordered, 20 mL of blood must be cleared prior to filling the blue-top tube.

- *Mastectomy* Do not perform a venipuncture from the arm on the side on which a mastectomy has been performed. A mastectomy causes **lymphostasis** in the arm. Lymphostasis is a lack of fluid drainage, and it may cause erroneous test results. In addition, lymphedema is a lifelong risk for a mastectomy patient. A venipuncture creates the potential for an infection or damage to lymph vessels. You should also refrain from performing a venipuncture on the side of axillary node dissection or radiation therapy to the axilla.

- *Hematoma* Specimens should not be collected from a hemotoma area. A venipuncture performed in an area of hematomas is painful to the patient and may cause erroneous results. Collect samples from an area without hematomas. If that is not possible, perform the venipuncture as far away as possible from the hematoma.

- *Scar tissue* Avoid performing venipunctures in areas of scar tissue. The tissue is difficult to penetrate with a needle and may be painful to the patient.

- *Fistula/cannula* Do not collect a specimen from a cannula or fistula.

- *Thrombosed veins* Do not attempt to obtain a specimen from thrombosed veins or veins burned by chemotherapy. It is very unlikely that an adequate blood flow will be established.

- *Edematous arms or hands* Blood samples taken from **edematous** extremities (those swollen with fluid) will provide erroneous test results.

- *Blood transfusions* Obtaining a blood sample from an arm being used for a blood transfusion may cause incorrect test results.

- *Burned areas* Do not perform a venipuncture in a burned area. The site is susceptible to infection, and a venipuncture would be very painful to the patient.

Assemble Collection Supplies

The evacuated system is the most commonly used system for collecting blood specimens. It is used primarily when collecting from healthy veins that are adequate in size to withstand the premeasured vacuum in the collection tube. The syringe/needle setup is used for patients with fragile veins. A syringe minimizes the pressure exerted against the vein wall when withdrawing blood. When you pull slowly on the plunger, the small vein is less apt to close.

The following equipment should be assembled, based on your preliminary assessment of the patient's veins:

- *Needle* Select the appropriate needle size, based on the patient's physical characteristics, the condition of the vein, and the amount of blood required.

- *Collection tube(s)* Select the appropriate color-coded tube(s) for the requested test(s), and the appropriate size to meet required specimen volume(s).

- Tourniquet

- Alcohol prep pad

- Gauze pads

- Needle holder for evacuated system
- *Adhesive bandage*   Select the appropriate bandage for the patient's needs.
- *Protective gloves*   Clean gloves are to be worn for each collection procedure.

PROCEDURE   # Performing the Venipuncture Using the Evacuated System

1. Securely thread the needle into the holder. An unsecured needle can fall out of the holder! Leave the cap on the needle to maintain sterility. Some safety needles come from the manufacturer with the needle attached to the holder.

2. Open the sterile gauze package. Leave the gauze on the inside surface of the package to maintain its sterility.

3. Remove the alcohol pad from its package and place it on top of the gauze. This prevents contamination of the alcohol pad.

4. Apply the tourniquet. This makes veins more prominent. Do not leave the tourniquet on for more than 1 minute (Figure 5-2A).

5. Put on protective gloves. Gloves reduce exposure to bloodborne pathogens.

6. Cleanse the venipuncture site with the alcohol pad by moving the pad in a circular motion from the center to the periphery of the site (Figure 5-2B). Allow the area to dry, or wipe it dry in an outward circular motion with a sterile gauze pad. Cleansing helps prevent microbiological contamination of both the specimen and the patient through the puncture site. Allowing the area to dry prevents hemolysis of the specimen and prevents a stinging sensation when skin is punctured.

7. Have the patient close the hand tightly to form a fist, making the veins more prominent. Do not pump the hand.

8. Remove the needle cap.

9. Inspect the needle to ensure that it is free of hooks and that the opening of the bevel is clear.

10. Anchor the vein. Grasp the patient's arm with your nondominant hand. The thumb should be placed 1 to 2 inches below the venipuncture site over the selected vein. Press down on the selected vein with the thumb, and pull the skin taut in the direction of the patient's hand. Your fingers should be underneath the patient's arm. The patient's arm should be in a downward position (Figure 5-2C).

11. Firmly grasp the needle holder with the dominant hand. Hold the needle holder with your thumb on top and your fingers underneath (Figure 5-2C).

12. Line up the needle with the vein. This lessens the possibility of puncturing through the whole vein, which can cause a painful hematoma.

13. Direct the bevel up. Positioning the bevel facing up allows for the flow of blood into the needle shaft.

14. Insert the needle into the vein at approximately a 30-degree angle, using a smooth, unhesitating motion. This angle helps prevent you from puncturing completely through the vein. A quick, unhesitating motion is less painful.

15. Hold the needle steady. Brace the holder firmly between the thumb and the underlying fingers that are resting on the patient's arm (Figure 5-2D).

16. Push the evacuated tube slowly forward onto the needle's other end.

17. Should blood flow not be established, take the following steps:

    a. Change the position of the needle. Press the tip of the needle slightly downward. The bevel may be pressing against a vein wall, preventing flow of blood into the needle.

    b. Pull the needle slightly backward. The bevel may have gone through the vein completely.

    c. Slightly rotate the needle to the left or right. The bevel may be against the vein's wall.

    d. Try another tube. The vacuum may have been lost in the first tube.

    e. Loosen the tourniquet to increase the flow of blood.

    f. Do not probe. If a second venipuncture is to be attempted, use a new setup that includes new needle and fresh gauze, alcohol pads, and tubes. If you are still unable to establish blood flow, withdraw the needle. Do not attempt a venipuncture more than twice. Notify the patient or the patient's nurse that another phlebotomist will be dispatched to obtain the specimen.

18. If a hematoma should form, release the tourniquet immediately and withdraw the needle, preventing excessive bleeding under the skin. Apply pressure to the venipuncture site.

19. Allow the blood to fill the tube. Do not change the position of the tube until it is withdrawn from the holder. Movement of the tube prior to withdrawal may cause a backflow of blood into the venous system.

20. If multiple tubes are to be collected, insert additional tubes using the correct order of draw (please refer to Figure 5-2):

   a. Blood culture tubes (this prevents any potential contamination of the specimen after multiple tubes are drawn)

   b. Blue (sodium citrate)

   c. Red stopper (no additive) with or without gel separator

   d. Green stopper (heparin)

   e. Lavender stopper (EDTA)

   f. Gray stopper (oxalate/fluoride)

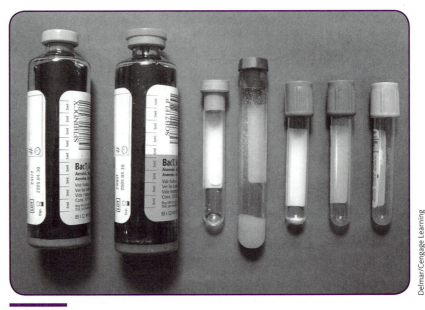

Figure 5-2 Collection tube order of draw.

Delmar/Cengage Learning

If additive carry-over from one collection tube to the next occurs, it may alter test results. The anticoagulants and additives can adversely affect test results. The EDTA in a lavender top tube contains salts of potassium. If the tube following the EDTA tube were to be a test for potassium, the potassium level may be falsely elevated. The patient with a normal potassium level may appear high and a patient with a low potassium may appear high. Therefore, a lavender top tube is drawn next to last in the correct order of draw. The incorrect order of draw can also impact coagulation studies collected in a light-blue tube. If a tube containing an anticoagulant is drawn before the light-blue top, the introduction of even a minute amount of anticoagulant will cause erroneous test results with a lengthened clotting time. The Clinical Laboratory Standards Institute (CLSI) no longer recommends drawing a discard tube when only a PT or a PTT is ordered. According to CLSI, a discard tube is not required when the citrate tube is the first or only tube drawn, unless special factor assays are being collected or when drawing through a winged collection set. Some facilities may still continue the practice of drawing a discard tube before drawing a light-blue collection tube.

21. Remove each filled tube. Immediately mix additive tubes by gently inverting them four to five times to prevent clots from forming. To avoid hemolysis, do not vigorously shake the tubes.

22. Instruct the patient to open the hand, thus decreasing venous pressure.

23. Remove the tourniquet, allowing blood circulation to resume. The tourniquet should not be on longer than 1 minute.

24. Prepare the gauze for placement over the venipuncture site, to act as a pressure bandage. Fold the gauze into quarters and place it lightly over the venipuncture site.

25. Remove the needle by withdrawing it slowly, being careful not to scratch the patient's arm with the needle tip. Activate any safety device.

26. Apply pressure with the gauze to the venipuncture site to prevent excess bleeding. Do not ask the patient to bend the elbow at the puncture site.

27. Dispose of the needle immediately to prevent an accidental puncture with a contaminated needle.

28. Bandage the venipuncture site. Continue to apply pressure until bleeding stops. Proper pressure can prevent hematomas from forming. Report any excessive bleeding to the patient's nurse, when appropriate. Patients on anticoagulant therapy or aspirin may experience prolonged bleeding. Take the time required to ensure that bleeding has stopped entirely before leaving the patient.

29. Label the specimen(s) in the patient's presence to ensure proper identification. Include the patient's name and identification number, the date, the time of collection, and your initials. Use the patient's identification band or the collection order to label the tubes. Never prelabel tubes prior to identifying the patient and collecting the blood sample. Do not accept unlabeled specimens collected by someone else with the intention of labeling the tubes yourself.

30. Complete special handling requirements to ensure integrity of the specimen. Some testing procedures require special specimen preparations, such as chilling the specimen or protecting it from light.

31. Complete clerical duties required by the laboratory.

32. Clean up blood collection materials. Make sure all equipment has been returned to its proper place. In the hospital, the patient's room must be returned to the order in which it was found. Return the bed rail to its original position. Turn off the light if it was off when you arrived in the room.

33. Discard used protective gloves to prevent contamination of the patient's area.

34. Wash hands. Gloves may have very small holes in them that cannot be seen with the naked eye.

35. Thank the patient, further enhancing a good customer service image.

36. Bag the blood samples and deliver them to the laboratory in a timely fashion.

Please refer to Figure 5-3.

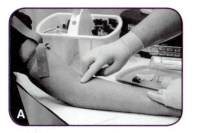
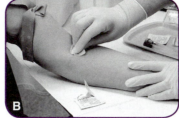
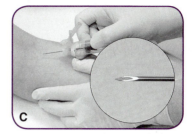

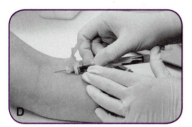
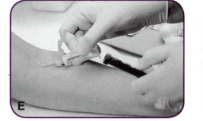
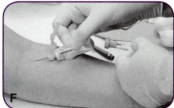

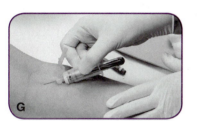
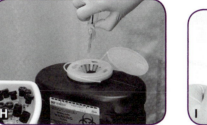
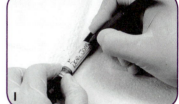

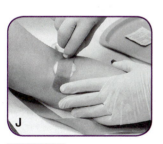
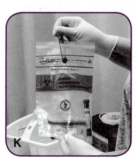
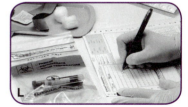

Figure 5-3 Performing venipuncture procedure with vacuum tube system. **(A)** Tie the tourniquet. **(B)** Prep the selected puncture site with alcohol. **(C)** Hold the skin taut and anchor the vein. Insert the needle with bevel up. **(D)** Push the collection tube forward. **(E)** Allow vacuum to fill tube. When tube is filled, remove while ensuring that needle does not pull out of puncture site. **(F)** Draw additional tubes if needed. **(G)** When last tube has filled, remove tourniquet. Withdraw the needle and activate safety feature. Apply pressure to puncture site. **(H)** Immediately dispose of needle into sharps container. **(I)** Label specimens. **(J)** Check puncture site to ensure bleeding has stopped, and bandage appropriately. **(K)** Package specimen for transport. **(L)** Complete necessary clerical duties.

Routine Venipuncture Using the Syringe/ Butterfly Needle Collection System

The procedure for using the syringe/butterfly needle setup is basically the same as for the evacuated system.

The butterfly or winged-tipped infusion device is most commonly used by the phlebotomist for blood collection from small, fragile veins. A 23-gauge needle is used most frequently. The device comes with a luer adapter for direct blood collection into evacuated tubes or with a female connector to be used with a syringe.

1. Greet the patient.
2. Identify the patient.
3. Select venipuncture site.
4. Assemble supplies.
5. Peel apart the package and remove needle device.
6. Thread the luer adapter into the holder. Check to make sure the adapter is securely in place.
7. If using a syringe, remove the tip cap of the syringe. Move the plunger forward and backward two to three times to ensure easy movement of the plunger. Remove the luer adapter. Securely attach the hub to the syringe.
8. Put on gloves.
9. Tie tourniquet.
10. Prep the venipuncture site.
11. Remove needle sheath.
12. Anchor the vein, and pull the skin taut.
13. Hold the needle by the wings, and perform puncture.
14. Pull back slowly on the plunger until an adequate specimen has been collected.
15. Remove tourniquet.
16. Quickly remove the needle and simultaneously press down on the puncture site with gauze.
17. Activate the needle safety device.
18. If using a syringe, gently pull back on the plunger approximately 0.5 mL to remove blood from tubing.
19. Remove hub from syringe.
20. Discard needle into sharps container.

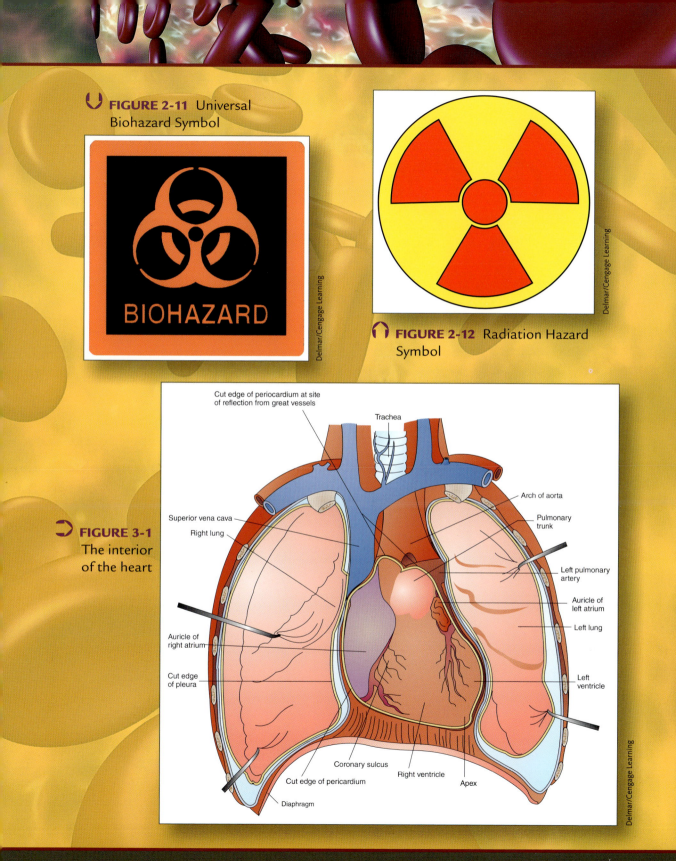

FIGURE 2-11 Universal Biohazard Symbol

BIOHAZARD

Delmar/Cengage Learning

FIGURE 2-12 Radiation Hazard Symbol

Delmar/Cengage Learning

FIGURE 3-1 The interior of the heart

Cut edge of periocardium at site of reflection from great vessels

Trachea

Superior vena cava

Right lung

Arch of aorta

Pulmonary trunk

Left pulmonary artery

Auricle of left atrium

Left lung

Auricle of right atrium

Left ventricle

Cut edge of pleura

Coronary sulcus

Right ventricle

Apex

Cut edge of pericardium

Diaphragm

Delmar/Cengage Learning

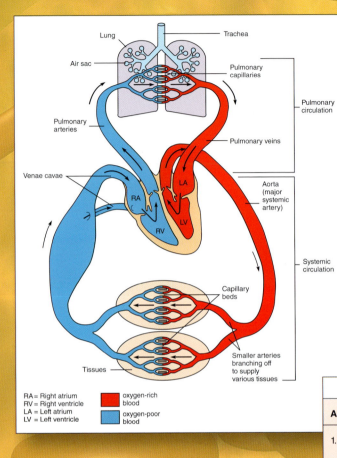

Lung
Trachea
Air sac
Pulmonary capillaries
Pulmonary circulation
Pulmonary arteries
Pulmonary veins
Venae cavae
LA
RA
Aorta (major systemic artery)
LV
RV
Systemic circulation
Capillary beds
Tissues
Smaller arteries branching off to supply various tissues

RA = Right atrium
RV = Right ventricle
LA = Left atrium
LV = Left ventricle

oxygen-rich blood
oxygen-poor blood

Delmar/Cengage Learning

◖ FIGURE 3-2 Schematic Drawing of Blood Circulation

◗ FIGURE 3-3 Blood Flow from Artery to Capillary to Vein

ARTERIES VERSUS VEINS	
Arteries	**Veins**
1. Carry blood from the heart, carry oxygenated blood (except pulmonary artery)	1. Carry blood to the heart, carry deoxygenated blood (except pulmonary vein)
2. Normally bright red in color	2. Normally dark red in color
3. Elastic walls that expand with surge of blood	3. Thin walls/less elastic
4. No valves	4. Valves
5. Can feel a pulse	5. No pulse

From Heart
To Heart
Artery
Arteriole
Capillaries
Venule
Vein

Delmar/Cengage Learning

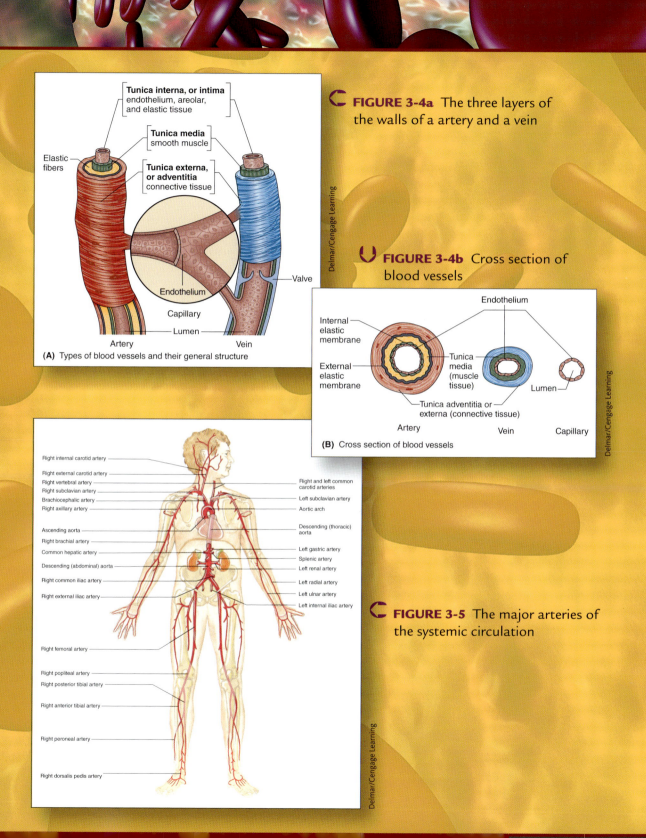

Tunica interna, or intima
endothelium, areolar, and elastic tissue

Tunica media
smooth muscle

Tunica externa, or adventitia
connective tissue

Elastic fibers

Endothelium

Capillary

Valve

Lumen

Artery

Vein

(A) Types of blood vessels and their general structure

Delmar/Cengage Learning

FIGURE 3-4a The three layers of the walls of a artery and a vein

FIGURE 3-4b Cross section of blood vessels

Endothelium

Internal elastic membrane

External elastic membrane

Tunica media (muscle tissue)

Lumen

Tunica adventitia or externa (connective tissue)

Artery

Vein

Capillary

(B) Cross section of blood vessels

Delmar/Cengage Learning

Right internal carotid artery
Right external carotid artery
Right vertebral artery
Right subclavian artery
Brachiocephalic artery
Right axillary artery
Ascending aorta
Right brachial artery
Common hepatic artery
Descending (abdominal) aorta
Right common iliac artery
Right external iliac artery

Right and left common carotid arteries
Left subclavian artery
Aortic arch
Descending (thoracic) aorta
Left gastric artery
Splenic artery
Left renal artery
Left radial artery
Left ulnar artery
Left internal iliac artery

Right femoral artery
Right popliteal artery
Right posterior tibial artery
Right anterior tibial artery
Right peroneal artery
Right dorsalis pedis artery

Delmar/Cengage Learning

FIGURE 3-5 The major arteries of the systemic circulation

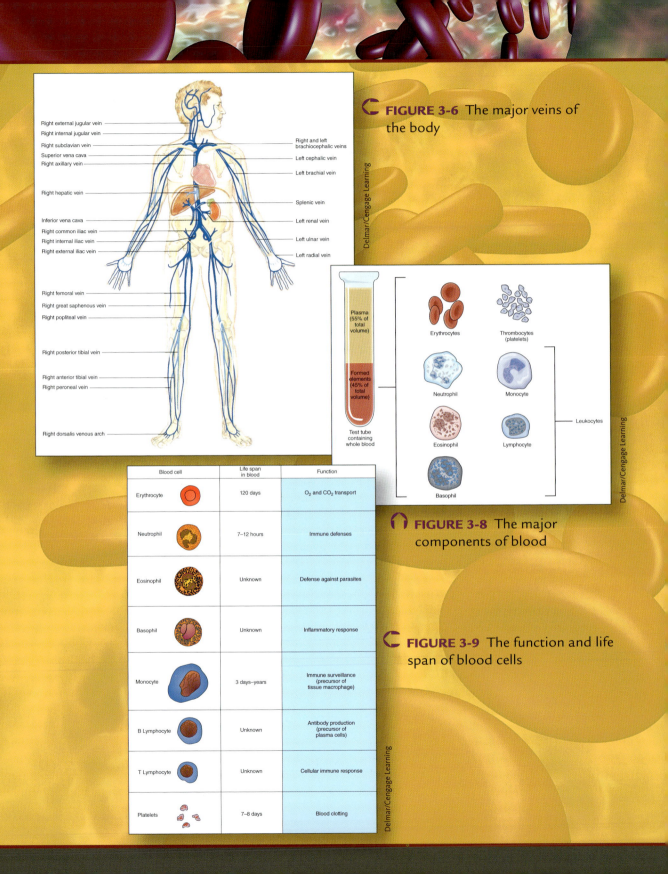

Right external jugular vein
Right internal jugular vein
Right subclavian vein
Superior vena cava
Right axillary vein
Right hepatic vein
Inferior vena cava
Right common iliac vein
Right internal iliac vein
Right external iliac vein
Right femoral vein
Right great saphenous vein
Right popliteal vein
Right posterior tibial vein
Right anterior tibial vein
Right peroneal vein
Right dorsalis venous arch

Right and left brachiocephalic veins
Left cephalic vein
Left brachial vein
Splenic vein
Left renal vein
Left ulnar vein
Left radial vein

FIGURE 3-6 The major veins of the body

Plasma (55% of total volume)
Formed elements (45% of total volume)
Test tube containing whole blood

Erythrocytes
Thrombocytes (platelets)
Neutrophil
Monocyte
Eosinophil
Lymphocyte
Basophil
Leukocytes

FIGURE 3-8 The major components of blood

Blood cell	Life span in blood	Function
Erythrocyte	120 days	O_2 and CO_2 transport
Neutrophil	7–12 hours	Immune defenses
Eosinophil	Unknown	Defense against parasites
Basophil	Unknown	Inflammatory response
Monocyte	3 days–years	Immune surveillance (precursor of tissue macrophage)
B Lymphocyte	Unknown	Antibody production (precursor of plasma cells)
T Lymphocyte	Unknown	Cellular immune response
Platelets	7–8 days	Blood clotting

FIGURE 3-9 The function and life span of blood cells

Delmar/Cengage Learning

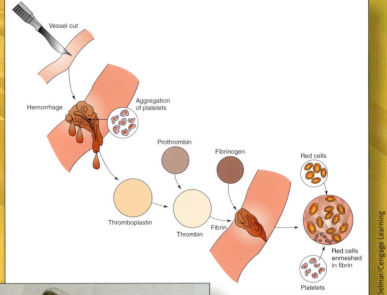

FIGURE 3-10 The stages of bloodclotting

Vessel cut

Hemorrhage

Aggregation of platelets

Prothrombin

Fibrinogen

Red cells

Thromboplastin

Thrombin

Fibrin

Red cells enmeshed in fibrin

Platelets

Delmar/Cengage Learning

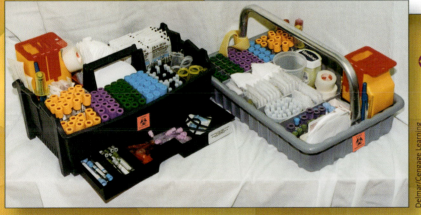

FIGURE 4-1 Routine Venipuncture Supplies— Part of a Phlebotomy Collection Tray

Delmar/Cengage Learning

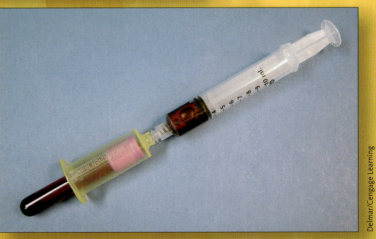

FIGURE 4-7 Blood Transfer Device

Delmar/Cengage Learning

BD Vacutainer® Venous Blood Collection

Tube Guide

For the full array of BD Vacutainer® Blood Collection Tubes, visit www.bd.com/vacutainer.
Many are available in a variety of sizes and draw volumes (for pediatric applications). Refer to our website for full descriptions.

BD Helping all people live healthy lives

BD Vacutainer® Tubes with BD Hemogard™ Closure	BD Vacutainer® Tubes with Conventional Stopper	Additive	Inversions at Blood Collection*	Laboratory Use	Your Lab's Draw Volume/Remarks
Gold	Red/Gray	• Clot activator and gel for serum separation	5	For serum determinations in chemistry. May be used for routine blood donor screening and diagnostic testing of serum for infectious disease.** Tube inversions ensure mixing of clot activator with blood. Blood clotting time: 30 minutes.	
Light Green	Green/Gray	• Lithium heparin and gel for plasma separation	8	For plasma determinations in chemistry. Tube inversions ensure mixing of anticoagulant (heparin) with blood to prevent clotting.	
Red	Red	• Silicone coated (glass) • Clot activator, Silicone coated (plastic)	0 5	For serum determinations in chemistry. May be used for routine blood donor screening and diagnostic testing of serum for infectious disease.** Tube inversions ensure mixing of clot activator with blood. Blood clotting time: 60 minutes.	
Orange	Gray/Yellow	• Thrombin	8	For stat serum determinations in chemistry. Tube inversions ensure mixing of clot activator (thrombin) with blood to activate clotting.	
Royal Blue		• Clot activator (plastic serum) • K_2EDTA (plastic)	8 8	For trace-element, toxicology, and nutritional-chemistry determinations. Special stopper formulation provides low levels of trace elements (see package insert). Tube inversions ensure mixing of either clot activator or anticoagulant (EDTA) with blood.	
Green	Green	• Sodium heparin • Lithium heparin	8 8	For plasma determinations in chemistry. Tube inversions ensure mixing of anticoagulant (heparin) with blood to prevent clotting.	
Gray	Gray	• Potassium oxalate/sodium fluoride • Sodium fluoride/Na_2 EDTA • Sodium fluoride (serum tube)	8 8 8	For glucose determinations. Oxalate and EDTA anticoagulants will give plasma samples. Sodium fluoride is the antiglycolytic agent. Tube inversions ensure proper mixing of additive with blood.	
Tan		• K_2EDTA (plastic)	8	For lead determinations. This tube is certified to contain less than .01 µg/mL(ppm) lead. Tube inversions prevent clotting.	
	Yellow	• Sodium polyanethol sulfonate (SPS) • Acid citrate dextrose additives (ACD): **Solution A -** 22.0 g/L trisodium citrate, 8.0 g/L citric acid, 24.5 g/L dextrose **Solution B -** 13.2 g/L trisodium citrate, 4.8 g/L citric acid, 14.7 g/L dextrose	8 8 8	SPS for blood culture specimen collections in microbiology. ACD for use in blood bank studies, HLA phenotyping, and DNA and paternity testing. Tube inversions ensure mixing of anticoagulant with blood to prevent clotting.	
Lavender	Lavender	• Liquid K_3EDTA (glass) • Spray-coated K_2EDTA (plastic)	8 8	K_2EDTA and K_3EDTA for whole blood hematology determinations. K_2EDTA may be used for routine immunohematology testing, and blood donor screening.*** Tube inversions ensure mixing of anticoagulant (EDTA) with blood to prevent clotting.	
White		• K_2EDTA with gel	8	For use in molecular diagnostic test methods (such as, but not limited to, polymerase chain reaction [PCR] and/or branched DNA [bDNA] amplification techniques.) Tube inversions ensure mixing of anticoagulant (EDTA) with blood to prevent clotting.	
Pink	Pink	• Spray-coated K_2EDTA (plastic)	8	For whole blood hematology determinations. May be used for routine immunohematology testing and blood donor screening.*** Designed with special cross-match label for patient information required by the AABB. Tube inversions prevent clotting.	
Light Blue Clear	Light Blue	• Buffered sodium citrate 0.105 M (≈3.2%) glass 0.109 M (3.2%) plastic • Citrate, theophylline, adenosine, dipyridamole (CTAD)	3-4 3-4	For coagulation determinations. CTAD for selected platelet function assays and routine coagulation determination. Tube inversions ensure mixing of anticoagulant (citrate) to prevent clotting.	
Clear	(New) Red/Light Gray	• None (plastic)	0	For use as a discard tube or secondary specimen tube.	

Note: BD Vacutainer® Tubes for pediatric and partial draw applications can be found on our website.

BD Diagnostics
Preanalytical Systems
1 Becton Drive
Franklin Lakes, NJ 07417 USA

BD Global Technical Services: 1.800.631.0174
vacutainer_techservices@bd.com
BD Customer Service: 1.888.237.2762
www.bd.com/vacutainer

* Invert gently, do not shake
** The performance characteristics of these tubes have not been established for infectious disease testing in general; therefore, users must validate the use of these tubes for their specific assay-instrument/reagent system combinations and specimen storage conditions.
*** The performance characteristics of these tubes have not been established for immunohematology testing in general; therefore, users must validate the use of these tubes for their specific assay-instrument/reagent system combinations and specimen storage conditions.

BD, BD Logo and all other trademarks are property of Becton, Dickinson and Company. © 2008 BD

Printed in USA   08/08   VS5229-9

⟩ **FIGURE 4-8**
Evacuated Tube
Collection Guide

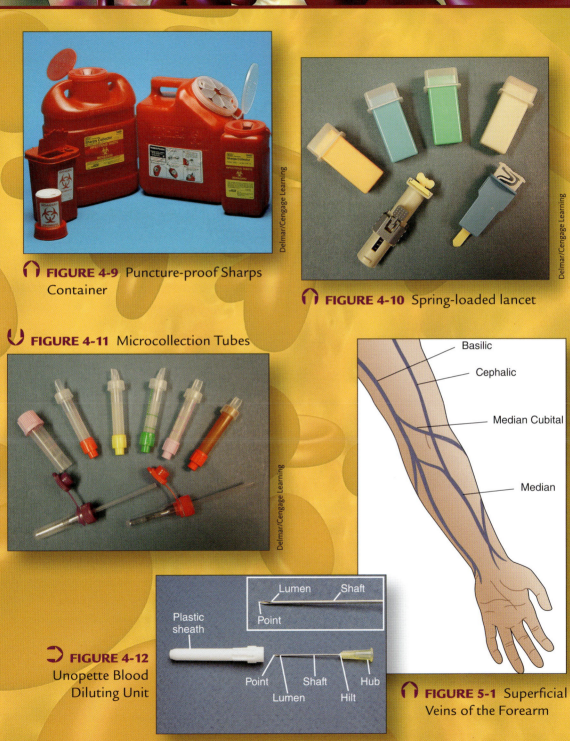

FIGURE 4-9 Puncture-proof Sharps Container

Delmar/Cengage Learning

FIGURE 4-10 Spring-loaded lancet

Delmar/Cengage Learning

FIGURE 4-11 Microcollection Tubes

Delmar/Cengage Learning

FIGURE 4-12 Unopette Blood Diluting Unit

Plastic sheath

Lumen   Shaft

Point

Point   Shaft   Hub

Lumen   Hilt

Delmar/Cengage Learning

Basilic

Cephalic

Median Cubital

Median

FIGURE 5-1 Superficial Veins of the Forearm

Delmar/Cengage Learning

FIGURE 5-3 Collection Tube Order of Draw

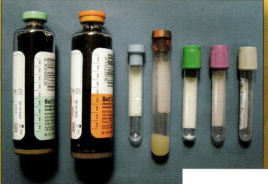

Delmar/Cengage Learning

FIGURE 9-3 Twenty-four Hour Collection Container

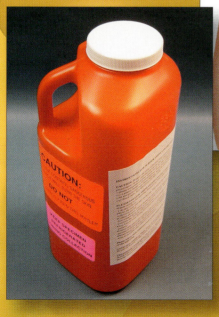

Delmar/Cengage Learning

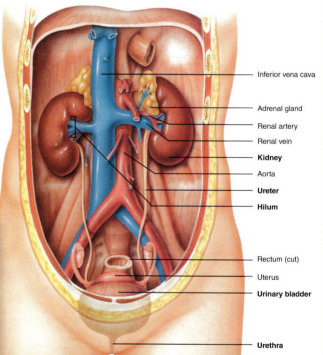

- Inferior vena cava
- Adrenal gland
- Renal artery
- Renal vein
- **Kidney**
- Aorta
- **Ureter**
- **Hilum**
- Rectum (cut)
- Uterus
- **Urinary bladder**
- **Urethra**

Delmar/Cengage Learning

FIGURE 9-1 Organs of the Urinary System

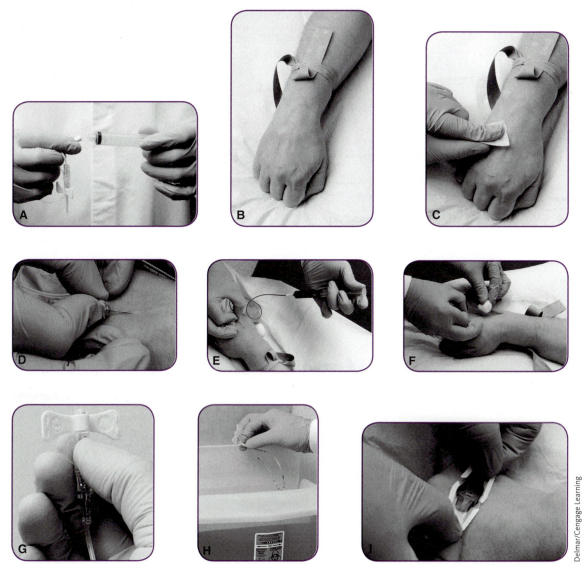

Figure 5-4 Venipuncture with the butterfly needle system. **(A)** Attach butterfly system to syringe. **(B)** Apply tourniquet with patient's hand closed. **(C)** Prep selected site with alcohol. **(D)** Insert needle at approximately 5–10 degree angle. **(E)** Slowly pull blood into syringe. **(F)** When the appropriate amount of blood has filled the syringe, remove tourniquet withdraw needle and apply pressure to site. **(G)** Immediately activate safety feature on needle. **(H)** Dispose of needle into sharps container. **(I)** Check to ensure bleeding has stopped. Apply bandage.

Delmar/Cengage Learning

21. Attach a blood transfer device.

22. Transfer blood into appropriate collection tubes using correct order of draw. The order of draw for a syringe is the same as for the evacuated system. Do not remove the stopper from the collection tube and manually fill the tube. Removing the stopper may allow for underfilling or overfilling the tube. In addition, there is a greater risk to exposure of blood should there be a spill. Do not leave the needle on the syringe and puncture the stopper. This increases the risk of an accidental needlestick to the phlebotomist.

23. Allow vacuum to draw blood into tube. Do not forcefully depress the syringe plunger.

24. Gently invert tubes 4-5 times to mix anticoagulant with blood.

25. Discard needle and transfer device into sharps container.

26. Label tubes with appropriate information, and bag for transport.

27. Bandage patient.

28. Discard gloves.

29. Clean up area.

30. Thank patient.

31. Wash hands.

Please refer to Figure 5-4.

■ SUMMARY

Careful blood collection techniques are critical for the phlebotomist. Organizing the workload, preparing the patient for the venipuncture in a pleasant manner, assembling the equipment efficiently, and performing a smooth, successful venipuncture are crucial aspects of the phlebotomist's work. Taking care not to injure the patient should also be foremost in the phlebotomist's mind, as well as ensuring personal safety during the blood draw. Experience will provide the phlebotomist with a smooth, efficient technique, both for communicating well with the patient and for performing a successful venipuncture.

■ REVIEW ACTIVITIES

1. Absolute identification of the patient is mandatory to _____
   _____.

2. ASAP orders have priority over _____ orders.

3. The hospital phlebotomist should awaken a patient before collecting a blood sample because _____.

4. The phlebotomist should not draw specimens above an intravenous site because _____.

5. A blood sample should not be collected from the arm on the side of a mastectomy because _____.

6. Specimens should not be collected from a hematoma area because _____.

7. The evacuated collection system should not be used on a small, fragile vein because _____.

8. Blood cultures should always be drawn first when drawing multiple tubes because _____.

9. Blood bank specimens should be drawn in _____ -stopper tubes rather than in gel-separator tubes.

10. When performing a venipuncture, the most frequently used veins in the forearm are the _____ and the _____.

11. A good, healthy vein feels _____ to the touch.

12. When selecting a vein, do not leave the tourniquet on the patient's arm for longer than _____ minute.

■ DISCUSSION QUESTIONS

1. You need to collect a CBC, protime, amylase, and BUN on a patient. After assessing the patient's veins, you determine that the best vein is on the right hand. What are the steps involved in collecting the blood specimen from this patient?

2. You enter the inpatient room of Mr. Smith. You find that he has no armband. However, you know Mr. Smith, because he was your high school science teacher. You are going to collect a CBC and B12. He has an IV in his right hand. What are the steps involved in collecting the blood specimen from Mr. Smith?

6 Collection by Skin Puncture

OBJECTIVES

After studying this unit, it is the responsibility of the learner to be able to:

1. List several situations in which the preferred method of blood collection is skin puncture.

2. Explain several situations in which skin puncture is not the preferred method of blood collection.

3. Describe the appropriate site selection criteria for heelsticks and fingersticks.

4. State the steps in performing a fingerstick.

5. Demonstrate the appropriate steps in performing a fingerstick.

6. State the steps to performing a heelstick.

"The differences in venous and skin-puncture blood should not restrict the use of skin-puncture blood."

—National Committee for Clinical Laboratory Standards (1986)

KEY TERMS

capillary action the process by which blood automatically flows into a thin tube during a capillary blood collection procedure

cyanotic displaying blueness of the skin, as from imperfectly oxygenated blood

interstitial fluid fluid between the tissues

lateral referring to the side

osteomyelitis an inflammatory disease of the bone, resulting from infection

plantar relating to the sole of the foot

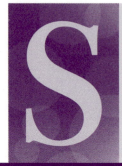

kin puncture, or capillary puncture, is a procedure in which the skin is punctured with a lancet to obtain a capillary blood sample for laboratory testing. While laboratory tests are most often performed on venous blood, there are situations in which venipuncture is not appropriate.

■ CHOOSING THE SKIN PUNCTURE

In several situations, the skin puncture may be preferable to the venipuncture. These situations may arise when:

- The patient is an infant, and a good vein is not found.
- The patient is a small child, and either a proper vein is not found or the child will not cooperate with the venipuncture.
- Tests are ordered that require only a few drops of blood.
- The patient is very apprehensive about a venipuncture and insists on a skin puncture (parents can also request this procedure for their child).
- Repeated venipunctures are not successful.
- The patient has severe burns.
- The patient has thrombotic tendencies.
- The patient's veins must be reserved for therapeutic purposes such as intravenous lines.
- The patient has fragile superficial veins.

A skin puncture is *not* appropriate when:

- The patient is severely dehydrated.
- The patient is in shock.
- The patient has chronic poor circulation.
- The patient is extremely cold.
- More blood than can be obtained by a skin puncture is needed for testing.

COMPOSITION OF SKIN PUNCTURE BLOOD

Skin puncture blood is different in composition from venous blood. Blood obtained by skin puncture is a combination of blood from capillaries, arterioles, and venules. It more closely resembles arterial blood than venous blood. Skin puncture blood may be used for laboratory testing so long as the technique is taken into consideration when interpreting the results of blood tests and when a small sample of blood is sufficient for the tests.

As the skin is punctured, tissue is damaged and **interstitial fluid**— the fluid present between tissues—is released. The first drop of blood will be diluted by this and fluid will need to be wiped away.

SITE SELECTION

A skin puncture (also called a capillary puncture) may also be performed on fingertips, heels, toes, or earlobes. However, the earlobe is not recommended as a site of choice, due to poor capillary access.

Children and Adults

Generally, the site of choice is the portion of the fingertip shown in Figure 6-1. Do not puncture the side or the tip of the finger. The ring finger and the middle finger are the appropriate fingers for puncture.

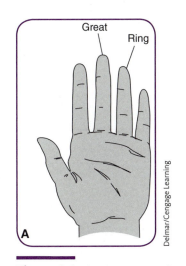
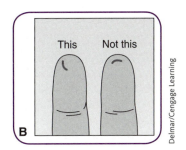

Figure 6-1 Finger puncture site.

The thumb, first finger, and fifth finger are not appropriate choices for skin puncture. The tissue on the fifth finger is much thinner than on the other fingers. The thumb and first finger are usually calloused. The nondonimant hand may be a better first option since the fingers may be less calloused. Patients requiring frequent fingersticks—such as for glucose monitoring, for example—should have the puncture site rotated. The puncture should be made perpendicular to the fingerprint. A perpendicular puncture will cause the blood to form a droplet. A parallel puncture will cause the blood to flow down the finger instead of forming a nice round drop.

Edematous (swollen) sites should be avoided, because a free flow of blood is impossible. Punctures in cold, or **cyanotic**, areas should also be avoided. Blood obtained from these sites may result in falsely high hemoglobin or cell-count values.

Infants

The site of choice is the **lateral** (side) area of the **plantar** surface of the heel ("plantar" refers to the sole of the foot). The darkened areas in Figure 6-2 show the preferred areas in which to perform a heel-stick. *Never* use the area of the heel bone as a puncture site. In addition, *never* puncture the area of the arch. Puncturing either of these areas may have serious consequences for the infant. Puncturing the heel bone may result in infection and **osteomyelitis**, an inflammatory disease of the bone. Puncturing the arch area may cause damage to nerves. *Never* perform a puncture that will go through a previous site. *Never* perform a skin puncture on the finger of an infant. The tissue on an infant's finger is much too thin, and the procedure could damage the bone.

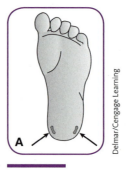

Delmar/Cengage Learning

Figure 6-2 Heel puncture site.

■ PREPARING THE SITE

A free flow of blood is important for accurate test results. Massaging the finger of the adult or child and the heel of the infant until the skin is pink will stimulate circulation. Warming the skin will also increase blood flow. A wet towel (or a packaged heating product) comfortably warmed to the touch may be applied to an adult's or child's finger or to the heel of an infant. The heat source should be applied for at least 3 minutes.

■ COLLECTION DEVICES

A wide variety of devices are now used to collect, process, and transport blood obtained from a skin puncture. Traditionally, blood is obtained with disposable capillary pipettes that resemble plastic straws. The blood flows into the tube through **capillary action**.

The process of collecting skin puncture blood has been simplified by the introduction of different types of microcollection devices. Figure 6-3 shows two such devices. These collection devices allow for easier measuring, color coding, stoppering, centrifugation, and storage of the blood samples. Collection caps, often shaped like a scoop, are used to collect the blood.

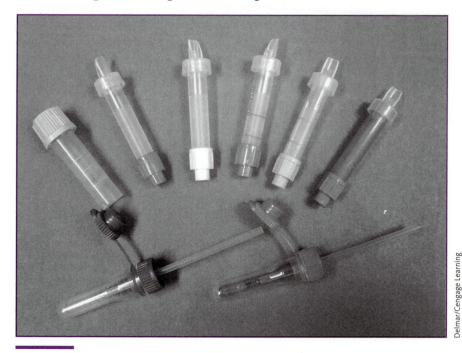

Delmar/Cengage Learning

Figure 6-3 Microcollection devices.

Lancets

A good flow of blood is obtained with the correct use of the skin puncture device. As with the collection devices, a wide variety of skin puncture lancets are available.

Lancets are designed to control the depth of the puncture so that no damage will be done to the site. Most lancets are either blades that the phlebotomist pushes into the skin or spring-loaded devices that lie on the surface of the skin and make an automatic puncture. The spring-loaded devices have a button that, when pressed, releases the lancet into the skin. Patients may be less frightened by this device, because they cannot see the actual blade penetrate the skin.

PROCEDURE   Performing a fingerstick

1. Identify and greet the patient. You must always be sure that the specimen is obtained from the correct patient.

2. Explain the procedure. The explanation should help to calm the patient and instill confidence in your ability as a phlebotomist.

3. Assemble the equipment: gloves, lancet or puncture device, alcohol prep pads, gauze, and collection device.

4. Select a puncture site.

5. Massage or warm the puncture site. The heel may be warmed with a warm cloth not to exceed 42°C (107°F). Commercial infant heel warmers are also available.

6. Put on gloves to prevent exposure to bloodborne pathogens.

7. Cleanse the fingertip with the alcohol prep pad to prevent microbiological contamination of the patient and the specimen.

8. Dry the fingertip to prevent hemolysis of the specimen from exposure to alcohol, and to reduce a stinging sensation for the patient.

9. Remove cover from lancet or other device to be used.

10. Grasp patient's finger, placing your thumb at the base of the fingernail. Wrap your fingers around the inside of the patient's finger. This maintains your control of the patient's finger while allowing you the best access to the puncture site.

11. If using a lancet, make a quick down-and-up motion with the lancet to firmly puncture the skin. One firm and quick puncture is less painful than a repeated puncture because of inadequate

penetration. Many beginners bounce the lancet off the finger instead of achieving penetration.

12. Dispose of the lancet in a sharps container. This prevents accidental puncture by the lancet.

13. Squeeze the patient's finger gently to stimulate release of one drop of blood.

14. Wipe away the first drop of blood with gauze. This drop of blood contains interstitial fluid that could dilute the sample.

15. Squeeze the patient's finger gently again, and fill the collecting device(s).

16. Collect hematology samples first to minimize the possibility of platelet clumping in the collection device. Gently tap the EDTA tube periodically to mix the blood with the anticoagulant. If filling capillary tubes or microhematocrit tubes, fill the tube approximately 2/3 full and seal with the appropriate sealing compound. These tubes may be labeled by wrapping a label around all of them and placing them into a nonadditive collection tube. Label the collection tube with the appropriate label information.

17. Slide your hand to the base of the patient's finger. Gently "milk" the patient's finger by firmly sliding your hand grasp back toward the patient's fingernail.

18. Do not squeeze excessively. This could result in contamination of the specimen with interstitial fluid. Allow the blood to flow freely into the tube. Do not "scoop" the blood into the collection tube. Doing so forces tissue fluids into the specimen.

19. When the collection device is sufficiently filled, place a clean, dry piece of gauze over the puncture site. Have the patient apply pressure until the bleeding has stopped. Do not use a bandage on the finger of a toddler. Young children may swallow small bandages and choke.

20. Mix all collection devices containing anticoagulant. This action prevents clotting of the specimen.

21. Dispose of all contaminated equipment, such as bloodied gauze, in a biohazard container.

22. Label specimen containers with appropriate information to ensure identification of specimen.

23. Remove gloves and dispose of them in a designated container to prevent contamination of the patient area.

24. Wash hands. Gloves may have very small holes.

ORDER OF DRAW FOR SKIN PUNCTURE

1. Slide for differential or stain
2. Blood gas or pH specimen
3. Hematology specimens (EDTA tubes)
4. Chemistry or other specimens (additive tubes first, then nonadditive tubes)

PERFORMING A HEELSTICK

Performing heelsticks on infants requires extra care and attention. (Please refer to Figure 6-4.) Selecting the appropriate puncture site is extremely important. Caution should be taken when applying pressure to the infant's foot. Do not puncture bruised areas or previous puncture sites.

Collecting blood samples in the hospital nursery requires the use of isolation techniques. Never take a collection tray into the nursery. Wash your hands thoroughly. This procedure may take as long as 3 minutes. Follow the instructions carefully for proper hand washing before entering a nursery.

Put on a long-sleeved gown and a mask, if required. Follow *all* nursery protocols for interacting with infants.

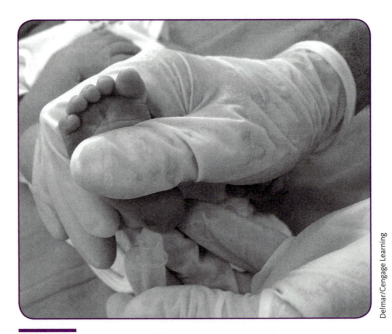

Delmar/Cengage Learning

Figure 6-4 Performing a heelstick.

PROCEDURE   Performing a Heelstick

1. Identify the infant.

2. Assemble supplies. Heelstick and fingerstick supplies are similar. However, a short-point lancet of less than 2.4 mm must be used for the heelstick. A puncture of more than 2.4 mm may cause bone damage. Open the gauze, alcohol prep, and lancet packages, but leave items inside the packages.

3. Put on gloves.

4. Warm and/or gently massage the heel.

5. Select an appropriate puncture site, avoiding previous puncture sites and the curvature of the heel.

6. Grasp the infant's foot firmly. A firm hold will help prevent sudden movement. Place your forefinger over the arch of the baby's foot and your thumb below the puncture site. Your remaining fingers should rest on top of the infant's foot. The baby's foot will be resting between your index finger and your third finger.

7. Cleanse the area with an alcohol prep.

8. Dry the site with clean gauze.

9. Puncture the skin in a quick, firm, down-and-up motion. Remember that the puncture should be perpendicular to the heelprint lines.

10. Wipe away the first drop of blood. This minimizes dilution with tissue fluid.

11. Fill the appropriate collection device(s). Collect hematology samples first.

12. When the collection device has been filled appropriately, elevate the infant's foot, place a clean gauze over the puncture site, and press firmly until bleeding stops.

13. Mix collection devices containing anticoagulant.

14. Label specimen(s). Mix-ups in identification may require another heelstick, which should be avoided in any way possible.

15. Dispose of contaminated equipment properly.

16. Remove gloves and place them in designated disposal units.

17. Wash hands.

A heelstick rather than a fingerstick should be used for children less than one year old. Children who are beginning to walk (and those up to the age of two years) should have blood samples collected by fingerstick, provided that an excellent vein is not available for venipuncture by an expert phlebotomist. Patients two years old and older should be considered candidates for a venipuncture.

[**ALERT**]

The phlebotomist must always use a short-point lancet on a baby's heel. A puncture of more than 2.4 mm may cause bone damage.

SUMMARY

Skin punctures, whether fingersticks or heelsticks, require much practice. Often the phlebotomist will be performing a skin puncture because the patient is compromised in some way. Skin punctures can be very painful for the patient, as well as time-consuming. Proper technique will minimize patient trauma, realize a good result, and take a short amount of time.

Drawing blood from infants takes much experience. Obtaining blood from a newborn in the nursery can be a very exacting task. Nurseries have strict rules to guard the babies from infection. The phlebotomist must be very careful to obtain the specimen without trauma to the baby's foot, and to collect a specimen that will give accurate results.

REVIEW ACTIVITIES

1. List five situations in which capillary puncture is preferred over a venipuncture.

    a. _____

    b. _____

    c. _____

    d. _____

    e. _____

2. List two situations in which a skin puncture would not be proper.

   a. _____

   b. _____

3. Skin puncture blood more closely resembles _____ blood than venous blood.

4. Capillary punctures may be performed on _____, _____, and _____.

5. The appropriate capillary puncture site on a fingertip is the

   _____.

6. The capillary puncture site of choice for an infant is the

   _____.

7. A heat source applied to the heel serves the purpose of

   _____.

8. The finger is not to be squeezed tightly when obtaining a blood sample because _____.

9. A heelstick rather than a fingerstick should be used for children less than _____.

10. Children who are beginning to walk should have blood samples collected by _____.

■ DISCUSSION QUESTIONS

1. An adult outpatient needs to have a CBC collected. The patient is very frightened about having his blood drawn. He has a good vein on right arm, but he refuses to let you draw from it. He states that he is in a hurry, and must get back to work. What should you do?

2. An 18-month-old child needs a CBC and blood culture drawn. You attempt a venipuncture, and are able to obtain only enough blood for the blood culture. The CBC is stat. What are your options?

7

Special Blood Collection Procedures

OBJECTIVES

After studying this unit, it is the responsibility of the learner to be able to:

1. Describe the procedure for performing a PKU test.
2. State the normal range values for PKU and bleeding times.
3. List the steps in performing a glucose tolerance test.
4. State the purpose of blood cultures.
5. List the steps in the collection of blood cultures.

"The basis of medicine is sympathy and the desire to help others, and whatever is done with this end must be called medicine."

—Frank Payne

KEY TERMS

aerobic living in the presence of air/oxygen

anaerobic living without air/oxygen

etiology the science and study of diseases and their causes and origins

hemostasis cessation of bleeding through the blood coagulation process

insulin hormone that regulates the metabolism of glucose

phenylalanine necessary for metabolizing protein amino acid essential for growth in children and for the metabolism of protein

septicemia the presence in the bloodstream of infectious microorganisms or their toxins

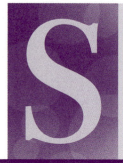

pecial procedures are necessary to collect blood samples for unique tests. Tests covered in this chapter are newborn screening, blood cultures, glucose testing, and bleeding times.

NEWBORN SCREENING

The purpose of routine newborn screening is to diagnose shortly after birth those infants with metabolic disorders for which early treatment will prevent or minimize serious, irreversible complications such as mental retardation. Newborn screening is cost-effective within the health care system, and can screen infants on a large scale. The tests that comprise the battery may vary from state to state. However, phenylketonuria and hypothyroidism testing are required in all states. These tests require blood collected from a heelstick onto filter paper.

Phenylketonuria (PKU) Screening

PKU is an inherited disorder of body chemistry that, if untreated, causes mental retardation. About one baby in 15,000 is born with PKU in the United States. The disorder occurs in all ethnic groups, but is most common in people of northern European descent.

PKU is a disease that affects the way the body processes food. Babies with PKU can't process an amino acid called **phenylalanine**, which is necessary for metabolizing protein. The phenylalanine builds up in the bloodstream and causes brain damage and mental retardation.

PKU was first recognized in 1934 by a mother of two mentally retarded children. She became aware that the urine of the children had an odd odor, and on the basis of this was able to have a biochemist, Dr. Asbjorn Folling, study the urine and identify phenylpyruvic acid. A test developed in the 1960s by the March of Dimes is used to screen for PKU. A blood specimen should be obtained from every neonate before the baby is discharged or transferred from the nursery. Any premature infant should have a specimen obtained for screening at or near the seventh day of age. Premature infants, infants weighing less than 11 kg (5 lb), may have elevated phenylalanine and tyrosine levels without having the genetic disease. This is probably a result of delayed development of appropriate enzyme activity in the liver. The test is highly accurate when performed when the baby is more than 24 hours but not more than 7 days of age. The child has to have a chance to ingest protein (mild) for a period of 24 hours. All states now routinely screen newborns for PKU.

Mental retardation can be prevented if the baby is treated with a special diet that is low in phenylalanine beginning before the fourth week of life. In a positive test for PKU, the blood phenylalanine is greater than 15 mg/100 mL. Testing should continue throughout an adult's life, and a diet low in protein maintained.

Hypothyroidism

Hypothyroidism results from an inadequate supply of the thyroid hormone, thyroxine. Approximately one out of every 4,000 newborn infants has hypothyroidism. Untreated, the child's growth will be stunted, and mental retardation will occur from lack of stimulation of the brain by the hormone thyroxine. Testing for hypothyroidism uses the same filter paper blood spots as for PKU screening. The condition is treated by utilizing thyroid hormone replacement treatment as soon as possible after birth.

PROCEDURE — Newborn Screening Procedure for Filter Paper Collection

1. Identify the baby.
2. Complete information on the specimen collection kit. Do not touch the area within the circles on the filter paper.
3. Assemble supplies.
4. Put on gloves.
5. Warm the heel. A warm, moist towel at a temperature no higher than 42°C (107.6°F) may be used to cover the site for 3 minutes.
6. Cleanse the heel with alcohol swab.
7. Air-dry the site, or wipe with dry sterile gauze.
8. Hold the infant's leg in a position lower than the heart.

9. Puncture the heel with an automated lancet device to a depth of no more than 2.4 mm on the plantar surface of the heel. (See Figure 7-1A.)

10. Wipe away the first drop of blood.

11. Dispose of lancet into sharps container.

12. Touch a large drop of blood against the filter paper within the circle. A sufficient amount of blood should soak through to fill the circle. Apply blood to only one side of the paper. Ensure that the blood has penetrated and saturated the paper. Do not layer successive drops of blood on the circle spot. Do not touch the blood spot.

13. Gently apply pressure with your thumb to form an additional drop of blood. Fill each circle. Do not squeeze the puncture. Doing so may cause hemolysis of the specimen and add tissue fluids to the specimen.

14. After the circles are filled, elevate the infant's foot, and press a sterile gauze against the puncture site. Please refer to Figure 7-1B.

15. Do not apply adhesive bandage.

16. Allow the blood spots to air-dry in a horizontal position. Keep away from direct sunlight. Do not stack or touch other surfaces to the filter paper during the drying process.

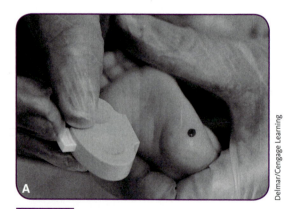
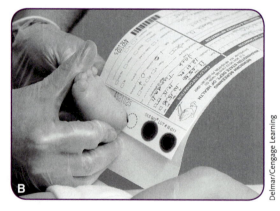

Delmar/Cengage Learning

Figure 7-1 Heelstick procedure for newborn screening. **(A)** Appropriate puncture site. **(B)** Apply drops of blood to circle on newborn screening card.

◼ BLOOD CULTURES

Blood cultures are ordered by physicians to rule out or confirm **septicemia**, a condition in which a microorganism has invaded the bloodstream. This condition can lead to the death of a patient.

The correct collection of blood cultures is extremely important. Because the results of these cultures lead to the identification of the condition's origin, or **etiology**, the phlebotomist plays a very significant role in ensuring the accuracy of this important test.

Blood cultures are usually ordered just before the beginning of antimicrobial therapy in a series of three draws. The cultures are collected in a series of three because that makes it more likely that the organism will be detected. In some cases it may be possible that the septicemia is caused by a localized infection. If this is suspected, the physician will order the series to be collected all at one time but from three different sites, rather than at three different times.

Blood cultures are drawn in sets of two bottles. One bottle is the **aerobic** bottle for those microorganisms that require oxygen to grow. The second bottle is called an **anaerobic** bottle for microorganisms requiring the absence of oxygen to grow. Please refer to Figure 7-2.

PROCEDURE Procedure for Blood Culture Collection

---

1. Identify the patient.
2. Select a site, and follow routine venipuncture procedure. Venipuncture sites do have an effect on the contamination rate among blood cultures. The antecubital vein is less likely to produce a contaminated specimen than the umbilical or femoral

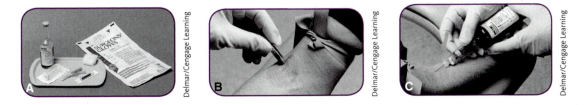

Delmar/Cengage Learning Delmar/Cengage Learning Delmar/Cengage Learning

Figure 7-2 Blood culture collection procedure. **(A)** Assemble blood culture collection supplies. **(B)** Prep venipuncture site with povidone-iodine in circular motion. **(C)** Perform venipuncture.

vein. Also, indwelling intravascular catheters are poor sources for blood culture collections. These lines become colonized with bacteria when left in place for longer than 48 hours. If a blood culture is obtained from an indwelling line, the femoral vein, or the umbilical vein, the source must be documented to ensure proper interpretation of test results.

3. Assemble the necessary equipment: culture bottles, commercial prep kit, alcohol preps, syringes, needles, gauze, tourniquet, gloves (refer to Figure 7-2A).

4. Reject any damaged or deteriorated culture vials.

5. Prepare the container(s). Swab the rubber stopper or diaphragm top of the culture bottle(s) with an antiseptic agent (iodine is not recommended for swabbing a rubber stopper). The stoppers may be contaminated and must be aseptically prepped.

6. Put on gloves.

7. Prep the venipuncture site. To aseptically prep a venipuncture site, 1 to 2 minutes must be allowed for the agent to have any effect. Scrub a 3- to 4-inch-square area for 2 minutes with a commercially prepared prep kit (Figure 7-2B). Allow the site to air-dry. Good technique requires that the puncture site not be repalpated. If absolutely necessary, the fingertip of the glove must be prepped in the same manner as the venipuncture site.

8. Apply the tourniquet, being very careful not to touch the puncture site with the tourniquet.

9. Perform the venipuncture and draw the appropriate volume of blood (Figure 7-2C).

10. Release the tourniquet.

11. Remove the needle and apply pressure to the venipuncture site with gauze.

12. If using needle and syringe, discharge any air that may have entered the syringe prior to injection. This allows the appropriate volume of blood to be added to the bottle.

13. Dispose of the needle appropriately in a sharps disposal unit.

14. Replace the needle with a safety transfer device.

15. Inoculate culture bottle(s) by adding the correct amount of blood. If too much blood is added, clotting may occur, impairing the recovery of bacteria.

16. Specimen requirements: 8 to 10 mL of blood should be injected into each culture vial. Fill the anaerobic bottle first. If using a winged blood collection set, fill the aerobic bottle first. The air in the tubing will prevent the growth of anaerobic organisms. Use a safety transfer device that pierces the stoppers of the blood culture bottles. If a fungus culture is ordered, 8 to 10 mL of blood is injected into the fungus culture vial.

17. Discard the needle and syringe in appropriate disposal units.

18. Label the specimens. Each label should include the site used for collection and the number of the sample, time collected, and phlebotomist's initials.

19. Remove and discard gloves in the appropriate container.

20. Wash hands.

21. Transport the specimens to the testing area.

ORAL GLUCOSE TOLERANCE TESTING

Patients with mild or diet-controlled diabetes may have fasting blood glucose levels within the normal range, but be unable to produce sufficient **insulin** for prompt metabolism of ingested carbohydrate. As a result, blood glucose rises to abnormally high levels and the return to normal is delayed. The glucose tolerance test detects a patient's decreased tolerance for glucose, and is most helpful in establishing a mild case of diabetes. The GTT is a timed test of blood and urine that determines the rate of removal of a concentrated dose of glucose from the bloodstream. In the healthy person, the insulin response to an oral dose of glucose is almost immediate, peaking in 30–60 minutes and returning to normal within 3 hours. Testing is usually done in the morning after an overnight fast.

Patient Preparation

1. The patient should be placed on a diet containing 1.75 grams of carbohydrate per kilogram of body weight for 3 days preceding the test. If carbohydrate intake has been too low preceding the test, a false diabetic-type curve may result. Drugs that may influence the test should be discontinued for 3 days before the test. Such drugs may include hormones, salicylates, diuretic agents, and hypoglycemic agents.

2. The test should be performed in the morning, and the patient must abstain from eating or drinking anything except water for 8 hours prior to the test. The patient must remain fasting for the duration of the test.

3. The patient should remain at rest during the test and refrain from smoking or chewing gum.

PROCEDURE   **Procedure for Glucose Tolerance Testing**

1. Draw a fasting blood glucose sample of venous blood. Also collect a fasting urine sample before proceeding with the test. Label the blood and urine samples with the patient's name, identification number, date, time, and phlebotomist initials. Write "Fasting" on the urine and blood samples.

2. Perform a rapid glucose test on the fasting sample. If the result is >140 mg/dL, delay proceeding with the test until a pathologist has been consulted.

3. Give the patient a glucose loading dose based on the following:

   a. Nonpregnant females and males over 100 lbs: 75 grams glucose.

   b. Pregnant females: 100 grams glucose.

   c. Patients under 100 lbs: 1.75 grams glucose per kilogram body weight.

4. Blood and urine specimens are collected at 1 hour, 1½ hour, 2 hours, 3 hours, etc, depending upon the physician order post-glucose ingestion. The glucose dose should be ingested within 5 minutes.

▓ BLEEDING TIME TEST

Bleeding time measures the primary phase of **hemostasis** (the interaction of the platelet with the blood vessel wall and the formation of the hemostatic plug). It is a test that involves the making of a standardized wound or incision and timing the process of clot formation. The bleeding time test detects vascular abnormalities and detects platelet abnormalities or deficiencies. A platelet count should be ordered before starting the bleeding time test. The bleeding time test should not be done when the platelet count is below 100,000 per cubic millimeter. There are three methods of bleeding time tests: Duke, Ivy, and Template or Surgicutt. The following procedure is for the Template Bleeding Time. Please refer to Figure 7-3.

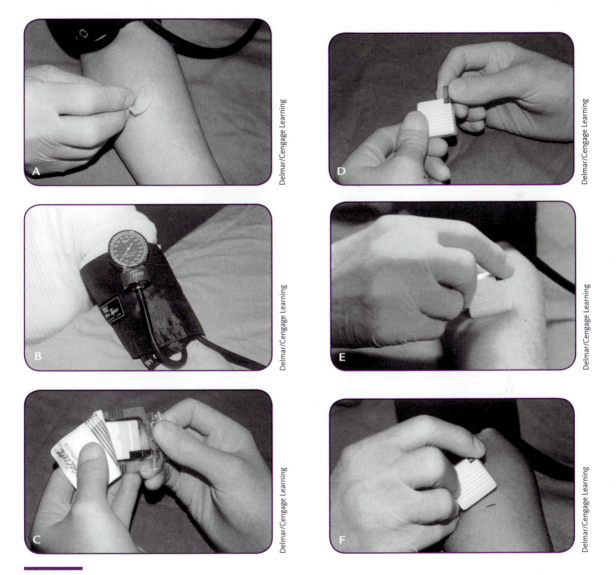

Figure 7-3 bleeding time procedure. **(A)** Prep forearm site with alcohol. **(B)** Place blood pressure cuff on patient's arm. **(C)** Remove blade from package. **(D)** Remove safety clip. **(E)** Rest device on prepped site. Push the trigger, and start stopwatch. **(F)** Immediately remove the device from the patient's forearm and dispose of device into sharps container. **(G)** Blot the blood with filter paper at 30-second intervals. **(H)** Continue to wick the blood every 30 seconds until no blood is visible. **(I)** Bandage the incision with a butterfly bandage.

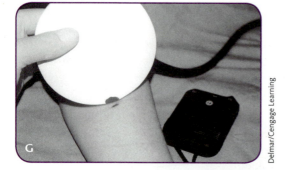

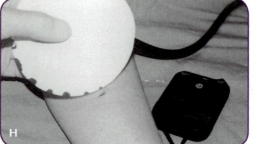

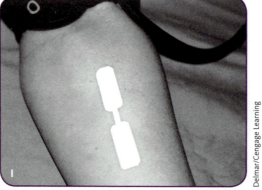

Delmar/Cengage Learning

Figure 7-3 *(continued)*

PROCEDURE Template Bleeding Time Procedure

The sterile disposable device used to make a uniform incision is a spring-loaded blade contained in a plastic housing. When triggered on the fore-arm or leg, the device makes one incision, 5mm long by 1mm deep. Simultaneously, a stopwatch is started. The blood from the incision is blotted at 30-second intervals. The time required for the bleeding to cease is estimated to the nearest half minute.

Materials

Single bladed retractable disposable unit

   Blood pressure cuff
   Stopwatch with second hand

Filter paper
Alcohol swab
Butterfly bandage
Gloves
Gauze
Bandage

Procedure:

1. Identify the patient using appropriate protocol.

2. Explain the procedure to the patient.

3. Obtain a drug history before the test is preformed.

4. Aspirin and aspirin-containing products will interfere with the test. The patient must be asked whether he has taken any such products within the last 7 days. Record all drugs taken on the patient history form.

5. Position the patient with forearm facing upward on a support. Select an area of the forearm distal to the antecubital fossa taking care to avoid surface veins, scars, and bruises.

6. Cleanse with an alcohol swab and allow the area to completely air-dry, at least 10 seconds (Figure 7-3A). If the patient has marked hair, lightly shave the area. Do not perform the test on an arm that is edematous, has an IV, or is on the side of a mastectomy.

7. Place the pressure cuff on the patient's upper arm, over the artery at the level of the heart (Figure 7-3B). Inflate the pressure cuff to 40 mm Hg. Hold the pressure for the duration of the test.

8. Place the unpackaged blade firmly on the forearm, being careful not to press down on the arm. Press the trigger to release the blade. See Figures 7-3C through F.

9. Dispose of the blade into a sharps container.

10. Immediately start the stopwatch when the incision has been made.

11. Begin to blot the blood every 30 seconds, being careful not to disturb the wound (Figure 7-3G).

12. Continue to blot every 30 seconds until the filter paper fails to wick blood (Figure 7-3H).

13. Should bleeding continue beyond 20 minutes, discontinue the procedure.

14. Stop the stopwatch.

15. Record the time in minutes and half minutes (example: 5.5 minutes).

16. Deflate the cuff and remove.

17. Bandage the wound with a butterfly bandage (Figure 7-3I). Cover with gauze and tape over gauze. Do not clean the wound with alcohol, which would remove the platelet plug.

18. Advise the patient not to disturb the bandage for 24 hours.

      Normal range: 3–9 minutes.

■ SUMMARY

It is important for phlebotomists to know the collection procedures required for unique tests such as newborn screening, blood cultures, oral glucose tolerance testing, and bleeding times. Correct collection of these tests ensures accurate test results necessary for physician diagnosis.

■ REVIEW ACTIVITIES

1. Blood cultures are used to rule out or confirm _____.

2. The purpose of newborn screening is to _____.

3. The two tests required in all states are _____ and _____.

4. A positive PKU is _____ mg/100mL.

5. A glucose tolerance test measures _____.

6. A glucose tolerance test requires _____ and _____ to be collected from the patient at what intervals?_____

7. A bleeding time measures _____.

8. The normal value test range for a bleeding time is _____ minutes.

■ DISCUSSION QUESTIONS

1. What factors may cause erroneous test results for blood cultures?

2. What is the purpose of testing for hypothyroidism in newborns?

3. Why is a medication history important in performing a bleeding time test?

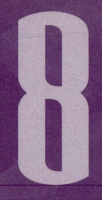

8

Special Considerations

OBJECTIVES

After studying this unit, it is the responsibility of the learner to be able to:

1. Describe how basic venipuncture techniques may be enhanced to accommodate the needs of infants.

2. List the different blood collection techniques used to collect specimens from infants.

3. State the different needs of children as they grow from infancy and describe how to adjust your approach to them when collecting blood samples.

4. Describe the various physical changes the elderly experience as they advance into later stages of their life.

5. Give examples of how the phlebotomist may adjust their interactions with the elderly to meet the needs of the patient.

6. Describe how venipuncture in the hand differs from a venipuncture in the antecubital fossa.

7. List the different types of vascular access lines.

8. Describe the collection of blood samples from vascular access lines.

"Care more for the individual patient than for the special features of the disease."

—Osler

KEY TERMS

central venous catheter an artificial line placed into the patient's body with the purpose of obtaining blood samples, administering drugs, supplying nutrition, and transfusing blood products

dorsal relating to the back side

heparin a drug used as an anticoagulant

patient-focused care an approach to health care in which services are simplified, decentralized, and placed close to the patient

point-of-care testing collection of a blood sample and immediate testing at the site of patient care

saline a solution containing sodium chloride used as a plasma substitute and a means to correct electrolyte imbalances

systolic contraction of the heart, the upper number of a blood pressure reading

tetany a disorder characterized by muscular twitching, cramps, and convulsions

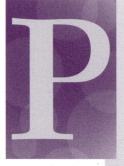

Phlebotomists must be able to apply routine venipuncture procedures to special situations. These situations require the ability to adjust to the needs of a particular patient. There is a need to understand the age-specific uniqueness of infants, children, and the elderly. Occasionally, patients have special needs requiring special collection procedures. Central access lines and point-of-care testing require collection procedures other than routine venipuncture.

▪ PEDIATRIC BLOOD COLLECTION

Both venipuncture and skin puncture techniques are used to collect blood specimens from children. The techniques are basically the same as those used to collect specimens from adults. However, children are not miniature versions of adults. They are unique individuals, and they require special consideration when the phlebotomist is collecting blood samples. These special considerations involve collection techniques as well as different interaction requirements for the phlebotomist. By performing the task well, the phlebotomist can help give children a positive image of health care workers.

Infants

Taking blood from infants is often intimidating to the phlebotomist. However, experience and confidence will make the phlebotomist as comfortable performing a venipuncture on an infant as on an adult. Infants have many needs, especially when they are ill. The phlebotomist can best satisfy those needs by observing infants' behavior and handling them in a soothing and reassuring manner. Different infants have different temperaments, and, of course, sick babies may respond in a very negative fashion. Research has found that babies can be classified as having one of three basic temperaments:

- Difficult—showing unpredictable patterns of response, intense reactions, and negative emotional moods
- Easy—predictable in response patterns and more positive in mood
- Slow to warm up—initially more like the difficult child, but not as intensively reactive.

While a phlebotomist may naturally be inclined to speak more gently to "easy" babies and to give them soothing touches, every effort must be made to give all babies their share of attention. Use a soft, soothing tone of voice to talk to the infant patient. Take time to softly stroke the infant's arm, hand, or foot before performing the puncture. Even though the infant is unable to communicate verbally, use your voice to make every effort to express feelings of warmth and concern to the child. Infants are human beings worthy of your full respect.

Blood samples may be collected from the infant by capillary puncture of the heel or by venipuncture if a vein is apparent. If venipuncture will be used, the **dorsal** hand vein technique is favorable, because it decreases hemolysis, decreases dilution due to interstitial fluid, decreases the number of punctures required, and decreases agitation of the infant (Jamieson & Hurwitz, 1994). To perform a venipuncture of the dorsal hand vein (a vein on the back of the hand), the procedure is almost the same as for a routine venipuncture, with a few exceptions.

PROCEDURE Dorsal Hand Vein Venipuncture

1. After putting on gloves, place the baby's wrist between your middle and index fingers and apply slight pressure. The pressure acts as a tourniquet to allow venous filling (Figure 8-1).

2. Lightly stroke the back of the infant's hand to help you see and palpate veins. Select only visible veins to avoid deep puncture.

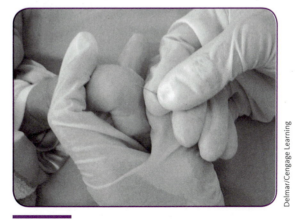

Delmar/Cengage Learning

Figure 8-1 Dorsal hand vein collection.

3. After selecting a vein, release the pressure of your index and middle fingers. This allows circulation to resume while you prep the site.

4. Cleanse the puncture site with alcohol by wiping in a circular manner, from the center to the outside.

5. Allow the alcohol to dry.

6. Reapply pressure to act as a tourniquet.

7. Using a 23-gauge needle with a translucent hub, with the bevel facing up, align the needle at approximately a 10-degree angle to the skin's surface and in a direct line with the vein. The alignment helps to prevent penetration through the vein.

8. Slowly puncture the skin and the vein. A rapid puncture may cause penetration through the vein.

9. As soon as blood appears in the hub, stop advancing the needle.

10. Leave the needle in place. This helps you avoid pulling out of or penetrating through the vein.

11. Allow the blood to drip from the hub into the microcollection tube.

12. If the steady flow of blood should stop, apply slight, intermittent pressure to increase blood flow. You may also try rotating the needle slightly.

13. Complete blood collection, and remove the needle.

14. Place gauze on the venipuncture site, and apply gentle pressure until bleeding stops.

15. Immediately discard the needle in a sharps disposal unit.

16. Label the collection tube with appropriate patient information.

Children

As children move from infancy to childhood, they begin to experience the need to become their own selves. It becomes very important for the child to succeed at "adult" tasks. The phlebotomist can demonstrate respect for child patients and build a positive rapport with them by allowing them to help in collecting the blood samples. For example, the phlebotomist may allow a child to hand over collection tubes, prep the arm, or perform a variety of other tasks. The phlebotomist can be creative in allowing children to participate, so long as safety is kept in mind.

Children tend to regress, however, when they become ill or they find themselves in stressful situations. Some children may regress back into infant behavior. This is normal, and the phlebotomist should not be harsh

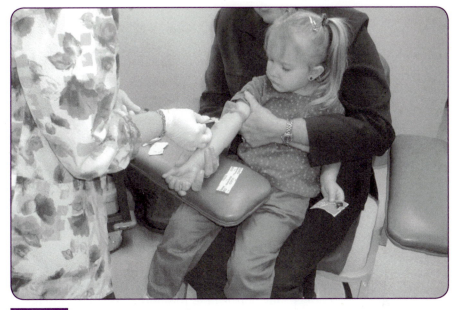

Delmar/Cengage Learning

Figure 8-2 Pediatric venipuncture.

or chide children for not acting their age. Instead, a more positive approach may be taken to encourage age-appropriate behavior. Describe the behavior you would like to see, and ask the child to help in "getting the job done." Talk to the child directly instead of talking "about" the child to the parent (Figure 8-2). Recognizing the uniqueness of the child as an individual, and understanding that the child is also a product of a developmental phase, will help you produce a positive experience for the child and the parent.

Often, especially when a child has a chronic or lengthy illness, brothers and sisters may be present when blood is drawn, whether the child is an outpatient or an inpatient. Brothers and sisters can be very close to the young patient and may feel excluded from that closeness when health care procedures are performed. Be alert to the presence and attitude of siblings. Include the siblings in the conversation. Ask them to assist with some small task, and give them the same "reward" stickers or toys that you give the young patient. This will help you and the family to work together to serve the best interests of the child who is ill.

■ ELDERLY BLOOD COLLECTION

Geriatrics is a medical specialty concerned with the prevention, diagnosis, and treatment of diseases in the elderly. Geriatric patients need special considerations, just as infants and children do. The effects of aging vary from one patient to another. However, we can make certain assumptions concerning the physiological aspects of elderly patients. Phlebotomists need to know these physiological considerations so that they can perform blood collection procedures more appropriately.

Several changes take place in the human body as it ages. Hearing and vision decline, muscle strength lessens, and soft tissues such as skin and blood vessels become less flexible.

Hearing Loss

The phlebotomist may need to speak slightly louder to an elderly patient. To test for hearing, ask, in a normal voice volume, the patient's name. If she or he does not appear to hear, you will know you must raise your voice slightly when speaking.

Vision Loss

The phlebotomist may need to assist with reading of information. The patient may not be able to see directional signs. The phlebotomist should be alert to helping elderly patients find different hospital departments.

Muscle Strength and Flexibility

The phlebotomist needs to practice patience when asking a patient to physically respond to requests. The elderly may need assistance in sitting up, adjusting arms for a venipuncture, walking to a drawing chair, and so on.

Skin and Blood Vessels

The phlebotomist must carefully observe the character of the vein prior to drawing a specimen. You may wish to use a smaller gauge needle, a butterfly setup, and so on. Elderly patients often have veins that collapse from the vacuum of the collection tube. Their skin is often fragile. The use of paper tape is recommended, or perhaps no tape at all. Taking time to apply pressure to the venipuncture site may be more appropriate.

Intelligence

A myth of aging is that intelligence diminishes with age. Studies show that there is relatively little decline in mental ability in healthy people at least up to age 70. However, studies also show that some older people may find it difficult to deal with many stimuli at once. In a busy outpatient laboratory, the phlebotomist must demonstrate patience and give the older patient time to respond to directions. There is also the potential for memory problems. The phlebotomist may need to repeat instructions.

Family Members

As the elderly become more dependent upon assistance from family members, be sure to include family members in instructions and directions. Explain to family members what is involved in the venipuncture, fasting requirements, and any other special instructions. Ask family members if they have any questions concerning the venipuncture and laboratory requirements.

ALTERNATIVE VENIPUNCTURE SITES

Whenever the phlebotomist is faced with the inability to find a suitable venipuncture site in the antecubital area, an alternative venipuncture site must be located. Venipuncture sites other than the antecubital fossa may include the dorsal side of the hand and wrist, the dorsal side of the ankle, and the dorsal side of the foot. Please refer to Figure 8-3 and Figure 8-4.

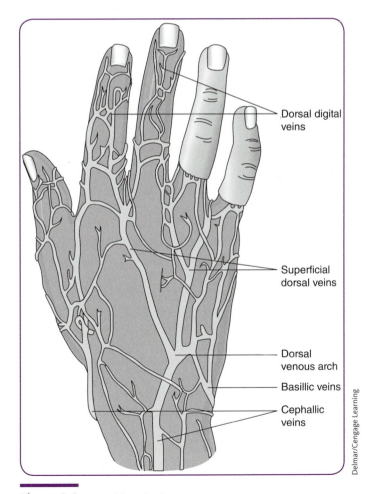

Dorsal digital veins

Superficial dorsal veins

Dorsal venous arch

Basillic veins

Cephallic veins

Delmar/Cengage Learning

Figure 8-3 Dorsal hand veins.

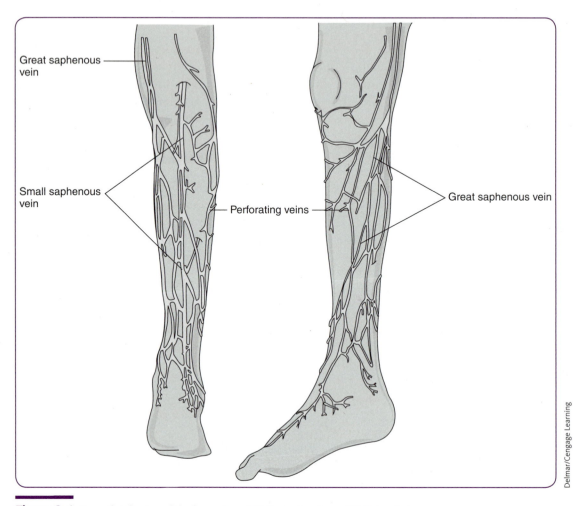

Delmar/Cengage Learning

Figure 8-4 Superficial veins of the lower leg. **(A)** Posterior view. **(B)** Lateral view.

Ankles and feet should be considered as a last resort. A physician's order must be obtained before puncturing a vein in the foot or ankle. Leg veins are very poor options due to the depth of the veins and the toughness of the skin. If the ankles and feet should be the choice site of a venipuncture, use a winged collection set with a syringe.

The dorsal site of the hand is often a good site for venipuncture. Adjusting the venipuncture technique will result in a successful puncture. The following adjustments from a routine venipuncture should include:

- The veins of the hand are more superficial than the veins in the antecubital fossa. The angle of the needle should be decreased to less than 30 degrees.

- Anchor the veins very securely. The top of the hand has less fatty tissue than the antecubital fossa. This means that the veins may roll away from the needle more easily than antecubital veins.

- Use a 23-gauge winged needle with a syringe. Use of the evacuated collection set will collapse the vein.

- Apply adequate pressure to the puncture site once the needle has been removed. Veins in the dorsal side of the hand are often fragile and may develop a hematoma when punctured.

- Never perform a venipuncture on the palm side of the hand and wrist. Tendons and nerves in the hand are close to the surface of the skin. There is an increased risk of injury to the patient.

■ VASCULAR ACCESS LINES

Central venous catheters (CVC) are indwelling lines that are used to administer drugs, fluids, and nutritional solutions; to make blood transfusions; and to obtain blood specimens for laboratory testing. Peripherally inserted central catheters (PICC), Hickman and Groshong Lines, **heparin** or **saline** locks, and implanted ports may be used to obtain blood samples for laboratory testing. The tunneled catheter is inserted into a vein at the neck, chest, or groin, and tunneled to an exit site underneath the skin. The exit site is usually located in the chest. The implanted port is similar to a tunneled catheter except that it is left entirely under the skin. The PICC is a CVC inserted into a vein in the arm instead of the neck, chest, or groin. Health care facilities have their own individual policies and procedures for obtaining blood specimens from the venous catheter. Phlebotomists or other health care personnel must have received special training before being allowed to utilize the catheters.

- A PICC is placed into the cephalic or basilic vein in the antecubital fossa. The tip of the line is threaded to the superior vena cava. PICCs can be used for weeks to months. Before obtaining a blood specimen, flush with 5 cc saline. The line must be cleared by drawing 5 mL of discard blood. Obtain the blood sample, and flush the line with 5 cc saline followed with 5 cc heparin.

- Hickman Line is silicon tubing placed surgically into a vein with the end tunneling through subcutaneous tissue to the exit site in the chest. The tip of the catheter ends in the superior vena cava. The catheter is for long-term use. The Hickman catheter requires a clamp to make sure the valve is closed. It is inserted into the jugular vein and then tunneled under the skin to the exit site. When a blood sample is being obtained, the line is first flushed with 5 cc saline. Discard 5 mL of blood. Obtain the blood sample and flush with 10 mL heparin saline. Sterile technique is extremely important, as the line may serve as an entry for pathogenic organisms.

- A Groshong Line is the same type of catheter as the Hickman Line. However, the flush does not contain heparin, and the discard blood should be 10 cc rather than 5 cc. The Groshong does not need a clamp. It has a three-way valve that prevents blood from backing up into the catheter. The valve opens outward during infusion, and opens inward during blood aspiration. When it is not being accessed, the valve remains closed.

- Heparin or saline locks are winged infusion sets that can be left in the vein for up to 48 hours. They are placed for the purpose of short-term use. They are often used by the laboratory for stimulation studies such as a cortisol stimulation test. The catheter is flushed with heparinized saline flush after each use.

Blood tests utilizing blood samples collected from central venous access (CVA) lines require special consideration. Coagulation studies should not use blood from CVAs. However, if absolutely necessary, 20 mL of discard blood must be obtained. The source of the blood must be documented. Please refer to Figure 8-5 and Figure 8-6.

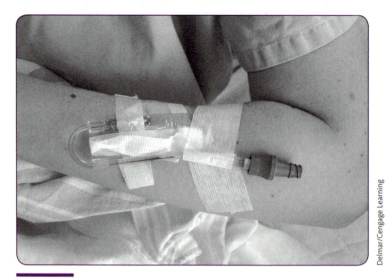

Delmar/Cengage Learning

Figure 8-5 Heparin lock.

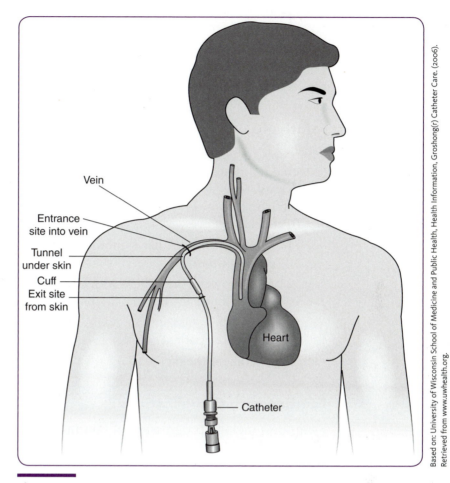

Vein

Entrance site into vein

Tunnel under skin

Cuff

Exit site from skin

Heart

Catheter

Based on: University of Wisconsin School of Medicine and Public Health, Health Information, Groshong(r) Catheter Care. (2006). Retrieved from www.uwhealth.org.

Figure 8-6 Placement of Groshong® Catheter.

PHYSIOLOGICAL VENIPUNCTURE REACTIONS

Prefainting Symptoms

Symptoms include increased nervousness, increased respiration, a slow and weak pulse, decreased blood pressure, pallor and mild sweating, nausea, and vomiting.

Treatment:

1. Elevate the patient's feet (or lower the patient's head if he or she is seated).

2. Have the patient inhale an opened ammonia capsule being careful not to touch the capsule to the patient's nose (test it before having the patient inhale).

   3. Apply a cool cloth to the patient's head.

   4. Reassure the patient.

   5. Instruct the patient to breathe slowly.

   6. Document the incident.

Fainting

Symptoms include moderate progression of the preceding symptoms, to include periods of unconsciousness, rapid and shallow respiration or hyperventilation, slow pulse, and hypotension with **systolic** pressure as low as 60 mm Hg.

   Treatment:

   1. Same as for shock-like symptoms without loss of consciousness.

   2. After arousing the patient with an ammonia capsule, give the patient fluids and instruct the patient to breathe into a paper bag.

   3. Loosen the patient's clothing.

   4. Document the incident.

Fainting with Complications

Symptoms include progression of fainting symptoms, including involuntary body movements, deeper loss of consciousness, and generalized state of **tetany**, rhythmic muscular contractions, raspy breathing, and cessation of muscle activity.

   Treatment:

   1. Notify the pathologist immediately.

   2. Follow the treatment for fainting.

   3. Document the incident.

Hematoma

There is bruising at the venipuncture site.

   Treatment:

   1. Remove and dispose of needle.

   2. Apply pressure for 5 minutes.

   3. Cold packs may be applied to reduce bruising and pain immediately after hematoma forms.

■ SPECIAL PATIENT CONSIDERATIONS

1. You may give the patient the names of any tests ordered. Do not attempt to explain why the physician ordered the tests.
2. Refer the patient to the physician for further explanation.

Patient Refuses Blood Draw

1. Do not argue with the patient.
2. Explain that the physician ordered the test, and explain any pertinent time considerations (if the test is a stat or timed test).
3. Ask if the patient still wishes to refuse the test.
4. If the patient refuses, report the objections to the nurse or physician, as appropriate.
5. Document the refusal in the laboratory.

Physician Is with the Patient

In a hospital setting, if the physician is with the patient when you arrive to perform a blood draw, ask the physician if the specimen needs to be collected at that time or if you should return later. The physician always has priority with the patient.

■ PATIENT-FOCUSED CARE AND POINT-OF-CARE TESTING

Patient-Focused Care

New opportunities for job enrichment are becoming available to phlebotomists. In the next several years, phlebotomists may have an opportunity to become part of the **patient-focused care** concept that has been initiated in several hospitals throughout the country. This concept implies expanded roles for phlebotomists and other health care workers.

Hospitals have begun to reassess their traditional approaches to providing health care. They need to enhance the quality of care while combining it with more cost-effective practices. Many recent studies show that the most obvious contributor to high costs and inefficiency is hospitals' poor organizational structure, which can result in multiple management layers, too many specialized job descriptions, communication problems, delays in performing procedures, and continuous disruptions for patients by a multitude of staff members from specialized units.

Greater continuity of care and reduced costs will be goals that hospitals actively pursue through reorganization. Patient-focused care is seen as one way to achieve those goals. Patient-focused care is a decentralized approach in which hospital processes are simplified to provide better inpatient services to the patient. It places routine services close to the patient. For example, instead of the phlebotomist's responding to the inpatient from a centralized laboratory, phlebotomy duties will be performed by multiskilled staff members assigned to the patient's nursing unit. These multiskilled workers may be nurse's aide-phlebotomists, ward clerk-phlebotomists, and so on. The objective is to broaden health care workers' qualifications so that the patient interacts with fewer workers and receives greater continuity of care. At the same time, costs and redundancy in services will be reduced, and response time in collecting blood samples will be greatly reduced. In addition, cross-training in other areas of health care will provide greater job satisfaction for the phlebotomist.

Point-of-Care Testing

Another aspect of patient-focused care is **point-of-care testing**. This involves the collection of a blood sample and then its immediate testing at the site of patient care. This site, or point-of-care, may be an operating room, an emergency room, a critical care unit, a physician's office, or the patient's own home. The purpose of point-of-care testing is to decrease turnaround time for blood tests. The new capabilities of testing instruments have made it possible to provide a very rapid response at the patient's point-of-care. Bedside care may include tests for glucose, hemoglobin, urine dipstick, sodium, potassium, ionized calcium, blood gases, and coagulation studies for managing heparin use.

New instruments developed for point-of-care testing are designed to make tests less dependent on the technical skill of the operator. This opens the door to a new area of training and to the expansion of skills for the phlebotomist. While many hospitals choose to use nurses as the test operators, some evidence shows that this is not the best solution in all situations. The hospital laboratory should always control the testing program. Nevertheless, medical technologists, nurses, and ancillary health care personnel may be trained to perform the tests. Each institution will make a decision based on its own unique requirements.

Many hospitals have found that nurses have so many tasks to perform that an added responsibility makes their work very difficult. In this case, phlebotomists may have an opportunity to perform point-of-care testing. Of course, the phlebotomist must be adequately trained, certified, and motivated to do the work. Phlebotomists must fully appreciate the seriousness of operator error. Studies have indicated that the most common problem behind testing errors has been lack of adequate training in operating the testing instrument and lack of practice with appropriate quality-control techniques.

While such innovative approaches to delivering health care will require some dramatic changes, they present an opportunity and a challenge to phlebotomists eager to participate in providing improved and cost-effective services.

SUMMARY

Procedures for specimen collection provide a very objective and standardized method for obtaining specimens. However, because of the nature of human beings, many situations arise that are not routine. The phlebotomist should know how to recognize these situations and respond appropriately. All events requiring special consideration must be documented and sent to Risk Management.

REVIEW ACTIVITIES

1. As children grow from infancy to childhood, they begin to experience the need to _____.

2. The purpose of point-of-care testing is to reduce _____.

3. The appropriate steps to take when an outpatient faints are _____.

4. Central venous access lines are used to _____.

5. Alternative venipuncture sites include _____, _____, _____, and _____.

DISCUSSION QUESTIONS

1. Describe the procedure for obtaining a blood sample from a Hickman Line for coagulation studies, blood cultures, a CBC, and electrolytes.

2. Describe how venipuncture technique for drawing from the top of a hand differs from a routine venipuncture in the antecubital fossa area.

9

Urine Tests

"Urine is a fluid secreted by the kidneys, transported through the ureters to the bladder, where it is stored until excreted from the body through the urethra. Changes in the color, acidity, and other characteristics of urine are important clues to many diseases."

—Mikel A. Rothenberg, M.D., and Charles F. Chapman

OBJECTIVES

After studying this chapter, it is the responsibility of the learner to be able to:

1. List the structures that make up the urinary system.
2. Describe the functions of the structures of the urinary system.
3. Discuss the function of the nephron.
4. Explain the major functions of the urinary system.
5. List and describe the different types of urine collections.
6. List the components of urine.

KEY TERMS

excretory organs organs that discharge wastes from the body

filtrates fluid that remains after a liquid is passed through a membranous filter

nephron structural and functional unit of the kidney

respiratory system consists of the nose, nasal cavity, pharynx, larynx, trachea, bronchi, and lungs

urinary system consists of the kidneys, ureters, urinary bladder, and urethra

urine fluid secreted by the kidneys

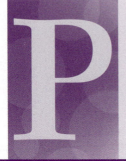

hlebotomists and lab technicians will be involved with collection, processing, and perhaps even testing **urine** specimens. The laboratory offers many different tests on urine specimens. This chapter will discuss the urinary system, the components of urine, and the procedures of the basic urine collection processes.

■ THE URINARY SYSTEM

The **urinary system** serves primarily to produce and eliminate urine. It consists of two kidneys, two ureters, one bladder, and one urethra. The kidneys are small fist-sized, bean-shaped organs located outside the peritoneal cavity on each side of the spine, at about the level of the last thoracic and upper two lumbar vertebrae. The right kidney is just below the liver and the left kidney below the spleen. The kidneys, the **respiratory system**, and the skin are the primary **excretory organs** of the body. The kidney's main function is to regulate the amount of water, electrolytes (sodium, potassium, chloride), and nitrogenous waste products (urea) from protein metabolism. Other functions of the kidney are to regulate blood pH, ion balance, and fluid balance. In addition, they assist in regulating blood pressure. Please refer to Figure 9-1.

The kidney is divided into an outer cortex and an inner medulla. The functional unit of the kidney is the **nephron**. There are more than 1,000,000 nephrons in each kidney. Each nephron is made up of a glomerus, which acts in filtering. In addition, a tubule is also part of the nephron. The tubule passes through the **filtrate**. Some solutes are reabsorbed, and others are secreted into the kidney for excretion. The glomerus is made up of a network of capillaries surrounded by a membrane called Bowman's capsule. This portion of the nephron is composed of the proximal convoluted tubule, the thin-walled segment, and the distal convoluted tubule. The thin-walled portion forms a loop called the loop of Henle. The collecting ducts join to form the papillary ducts, which empty at the tips of the papillae into the calyces. The filtrate drains into the renal pelvis. The filtrate now is urine. Urine passes from the pelvis of the kidney down the ureter and into the bladder.

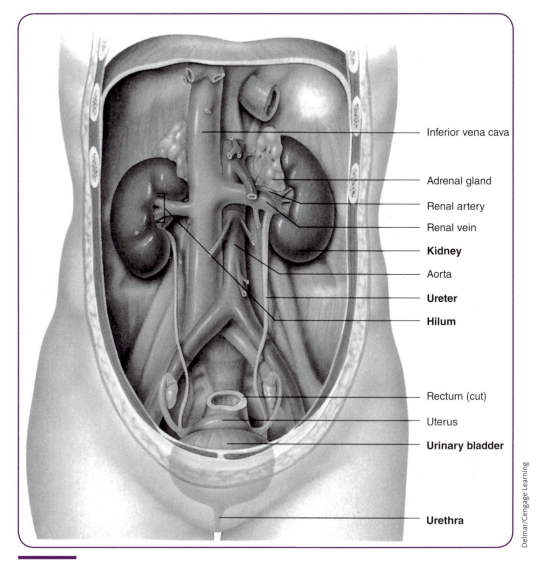

Inferior vena cava

Adrenal gland

Renal artery

Renal vein

Kidney

Aorta

Ureter

Hilum

Rectum (cut)

Uterus

Urinary bladder

Urethra

Delmar/Cengage Learning

Figure 9-1 Organs of the urinary system.

   The ureters are small tubes that carry urine from the renal pelvis to the posterior inferior portion of the urinary bladder. The urinary bladder is a hollow muscular container that lies in the pelvic cavity just posterior to the pubic symphysis. The bladder functions to store urine, and the size of the bladder depends on the quantity of urine present. The urine remains in the bladder until it is voided through the urethra. The bladder can hold from a few milliliters to a maximum of 1000 milliliters. The urethra is a tube that exits the bladder near the entrance of the two ureters. The urethra carries urine from the bladder to the outside of the body.

■ URINE

Urine contains thousands of dissolved substances, although the three principal constituents are water, urea, and sodium chloride. More solids are excreted from the body in urine than by any other process. The composition of urine depends greatly on the quality and the quantity of the excreted waste material. Almost all the substances found in urine are also found in blood, although in different concentrations. The largest component of urine is water. The majority of solutes are urea, chloride, sodium, potassium, phosphate, sulfate, creatinine, and uric acid.

■ URINE COLLECTION

Urine Containers

One of the most important aspects of urine collection is the container. It is very important that the container be clean. The laboratory should supply the container for the patient's collection. Disposable, nonsterile, plastic containers are the most common. The containers come in various sizes and must have tight-fitting lids. Pliable polyethylene bags with adhesive are used for collection of urine from infants. For specimens that are to be collected over a period of time, as in a 24-hour collection, large, wide-mouthed plastic containers are used. Sterile plastic containers are used when the urine is to be cultured for bacteria. Please refer to Figure 9-2 and Figure 9-3.

Give the patient the following instructions for collecting a urine specimen.

Random or Spot Specimen

The patient may void at any time of the day or night and collect a portion of the urine in a clean container.

Fasting Specimen

The patient will void four or more hours following the ingestion of food and discard the specimen. The patient will collect the next voided specimen, which can be regarded as a fasting specimen. Refrigerate the specimen until it is transported to the laboratory.

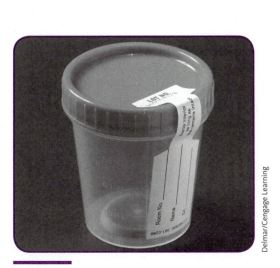

Delmar/Cengage Learning

Figure 9-2 One-time urine collection container.

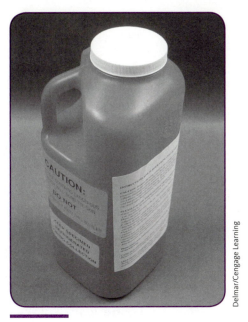

Delmar/Cengage Learning

Figure 9-3 Twenty-four-hour collection container.

First Morning Specimen

The patient will void before going to sleep for the evening and discard the specimen. When getting up, the patient will collect the urine specimen, which is identified as first morning specimen. The first specimen is more concentrated and may contain small amounts of abnormal elements. First morning specimens are preferred for screening for bacteria because they provide incubation time necessary for multiplying bacteria.

Midstream Specimen

The patient will begin to urinate in the toilet. When approximately half of the voiding is completed, without interrupting the process of urination, the patient will collect a portion of urine in the container, and then pass the last portion of urine flow into the toilet.

Clean-Catch Specimen

The external genitalia are washed by the patient using a mild antiseptic solution. A midstream specimen is then collected in a clean container.

Give the patient the following instructions for cleansing the genital area:

Men

1. If you are not circumcised, draw back the foreskin before cleansing.
2. Clean the tip of the penis using a sterile cleansing towelette, beginning at the tip and moving toward the base. Repeat the cleansing process using a second towelette.

Women

1. Squat over the toilet and use the fingers of one hand to separate and hold open the folds of the skin in the genital area.
2. Clean the urinary opening and surrounding area with a sterile cleansing towelette, moving from front to back. Repeat.

PROCEDURE Timed-Collection Urine Specimen

1. Obtain a large-mouth plastic container from the laboratory.
2. Have the patient void completely and discard the specimen.
3. Note the time, and collect all urine voided thereafter until the end of the collection time. Have the patient void completely at the end of the collection time and save the final specimen, adding it to the previously voided specimen.
4. Keep the urine collection on ice or refrigerated until the collection time is completed.

If any urine during the collection time is lost accidentally due to spillage, leakage, or loss with a bowel movement, the collection must be terminated and begun again at the start of the process.

During the time of collection, individual specimens should not be removed for routine urinalysis, glucose tolerance urines, etc. The entire amount of all the voided specimens must be pooled together and submitted to the laboratory.

Urine Culture Collection

A urine specimen is collected by the patient using the clean-catch mid-stream collection procedure. The urine container must be a sterile container. The specimen must be cultured within one hour of collection.

■ SUMMARY

If urinalysis is to provide accurate test results, it is mandatory that attention be given to proper specimen handling and preservation. Examination of a fresh specimen is very important. Because urine is unstable, changes begin to occur in a voided specimen, which may cause misleading results. As urine decomposes, glucose decreases, bilirubin decreases, and other chemical reactions occur. If a urine specimen cannot be examined within two hours, the specimen should be refrigerated.

■ REVIEW ACTIVITIES

1. The urinary system is composed of _____
_____.

2. Urine components include _____
_____.

3. The major three functions of the urinary system are:

a. _____

b. _____

c. _____

■ DISCUSSION QUESTIONS

1. Describe the different factors that can produce erroneous test results in urine testing.

2. Discuss the functions of the urinary system.

3. Describe the urine collection procedure for:

a. Random specimen

b. Fasting specimen

c. Midstream specimen

d. Clean-catch specimen

e. Timed-collection specimen

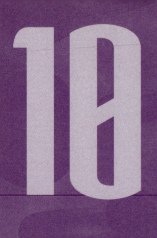

18

Common Laboratory Tests

OBJECTIVES

After studying this unit, it is the responsibility of the learner to be able to:

1. Discuss the most common laboratory tests and explain why they might be ordered.

2. Name the appropriate collection tubes for the most common laboratory tests.

3. Discuss abnormal test results for the most common laboratory tests.

"*The role of the laboratory in diagnosis and treatment continues to gain importance as newer tests and analytic methods allow diagnoses that were not possible before. Clinicians increasingly depend on laboratory test data.*"

—Jacques Wallach, M.D.

KEY TERMS

atherosclerosis a disease in which arteries are severely narrowed by lipid deposits on the inner walls

bile a yellow or greenish liquid secreted by the liver that aids in digestion

bilirubin a reddish-yellow pigment in urine, blood, or bile

cirrhosis inflammation of an organ, particularly the liver

colitis inflammation of the colon

enzymes protein substances produced by living cells; they are essential to life, as they act as catalysts in metabolism

occult hidden

urobilinogen compound formed in the intestine from the breakdown of bilirubin

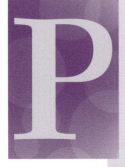

Phlebotomists are not responsible for ordering tests or interpreting laboratory test results. However, a general knowledge of laboratory tests and what constitutes a normal result is helpful.

Laboratory tests are delegated for testing to specific departments. Such delegation may differ among health care facilities. For instance, a urinalysis may be performed in the hematology department in one laboratory and the chemistry department in another. Specimen collection requirements can also vary among laboratories. This chapter will review collection requirements and normal test values for 50 of the most common laboratory tests, as well as some of the reasons a physician may order the tests. Normal-value ranges may vary slightly, depending on the testing methods used in individual laboratories. Collection tube requirements also may vary.

■ 50 COMMON TESTS

ABO

Collection tube: red top

The ABO (blood typing) test is used to determine the blood type (A, B, or O) of all blood donors and all potential blood recipients. Patients who need blood must receive blood products that are compatible with their own blood group. Surgical patients are typed prior to surgery.

Acid Phosphatase (ACP)

Collection tube: red top
Normal values:
    Men: 0.5–11.7 units/L
    Women: 0.3–9.2 units/L

Acid phosphatase is an **enzyme** that is widely distributed in tissue. A significant concentration of acid phosphatase is found in the prostate gland in men. The test is used to diagnose metastatic cancer of the prostate and to follow the effectiveness of treatment. Acid phosphatase is also present in high concentrations in seminal fluid, and this test may be ordered in an investigation of rape. Moderately elevated levels may also occur with any cancer that has metastasized to the bone, hepatitis, acute renal failure, and sickle cell crisis.

Activated Partial Thromboplastin Time (APTT)

Collection tube: blue top
Normal values: 30–45 sec

The APTT is a screening test for coagulation disorders. It is important for monitoring heparin therapy.

Alanine Aminotransferase (ALT)

Collection tube: red top
Normal values: 2–45 units/L

This test (formerly called SGPT) evaluates enzyme levels, primarily to diagnose liver disease.

Alcohol (Ethyl, Legal, or Medical)

Collection tube: red top
Normal values: none detected

Testing is done to detect the presence of alcohol, to indicate overdose or alcohol-impaired driving.

Aldolase

Collection tube: red top
Normal values: 1.5–12.0 units/L

Aldolase is a glycolytic enzyme that catalyzes the breakdown of glucose. It is used in diagnostic situations where acute hepatitis, muscular atrophy, myocardial infarction, or malignancy is suspected.

Alkaline Phosphatase (ALP)

Collection tube: red top
Normal values:
    Adult: 20–70 units/L
    Child: 20–150 units/L

ALP is an enzyme originating mainly in the bone, the liver, and the placenta. It is used as a tumor marker and an index of liver and bone disease.

Ammonia

Collection tube: 10 mL green top. Pack in ice
Normal values: <50 mcg/dL

Ammonia is a nonprotein nitrogen compound that helps maintain acid-base balance. Normally, the body uses the nitrogen fraction of ammonia to rebuild amino acids. It then converts the ammonia to urea in the liver for excretion by the kidneys. In liver diseases, ammonia can bypass the liver and accumulate in the blood. A test for ammonia levels is ordered to monitor the progression of severe hepatic disease and the effectiveness of therapy.

Amylase

Collection tube: red top
Normal values: 50–150 units/L

Amylase is an enzyme that is produced by the pancreas, salivary glands, liver, and fallopian tubes. It changes starch to sugar. If there is an inflammation of the pancreas or salivary glands, there is an increased level of this enzyme. Increased levels may also occur in mumps, alcohol poisoning, ruptured tubal pregnancy, and cholecystitis (inflammation of the gallbladder).

Antinuclear Antibody (ANA)

Collection tube: red top
Normal values: negative

An ANA test is used to diagnose autoimmune diseases, such as lupus erythematosus (SLE), scleroderma, and rheumatoid arthritis.

Arterial Blood Gases

Specimen type: Arterial blood obtained by special collection.

The purpose of the test is to assess the adequacy of oxygenation, assess the adequacy of ventilation, and assess the acid-base status by measuring the respiratory and nonrespiratory components. Arterial blood gases are used to monitor critically ill patients, to establish baseline values in the perioperative period, to follow up postoperative patients in the detection and treatment of electrolyte imbalances, and in conjunction with pulmonary function testing.

Aspartate Aminotransferase (AST)

Collection tube: red top
Normal values
>Men: 27–47 units/L
>Women: 5–55 units/L

AST is an enzyme (formerly called SGOT) that is released into the circulation following the injury or death of cells in tissues of high metabolic activity. Following a severe injury, the enzyme level will rise in 12 hours and remain elevated for about 5 days. In the case of myocardial infarction, the enzyme may be increased to 4 to 10 times its normal value. Liver disease also elevates the level, to 10 to 100 times the normal level.

Bilirubin

Collection tube: red top
Normal values:
>Total: 0.2–1.0 mg/dL
>Conjugated: 0.0–0.2 mg/dL
>Indirect unconjugated: 0.2–0.8 mg/dL
>Newborn: 1.5–12.0 mg/dL

Bilirubin is a by-product of hemolysis. The reddish-yellow pigment is removed from the body by the liver through the excretion of **bile**, a fluid that aids in digestion. A rise in serum levels can occur if there is excessive destruction of red blood cells or if the liver is unable to excrete the normal amounts of bilirubin. A normal level of total bilirubin rules out impairment of the excretory function of the liver or excessive hemolysis of red cells. Excessive amounts of bilirubin give the yellow hue to the skin that is a sign of jaundice. In newborns, critical levels of bilirubin call for aggressive treatment to prevent mental retardation.

Bleeding Time (Duke and Ivy Methods)

Collection tube: special procedure
Normal values: 3–10 min

Bleeding time measures the interaction of platelets with the blood vessel wall and the formation of a clot. It is used to detect vascular abnormalities and platelet abnormalities or deficiencies.

Blood Culture

Collection tube: broth culture bottles
Normal values: no growth

Blood cultures are used to detect septicemia.

Blood Urea Nitrogen (BUN)

Collection tube: green or red top
Normal values:
    Adult: 7–18 mg/dL
    Child: 5–18 mg/dL

Urea is formed in the liver. It is carried to the kidneys by the blood, to be excreted in the urine. A BUN test measures the nitrogen portion of urea. The most common cause of elevated BUN levels is inadequate excretion of urea due to kidney or urinary obstruction. Inadequate excretion may occur with shock, dehydration, gastrointestinal hemorrhage, infection diabetes, some malignancies, acute myocardial infarction, chronic gout, and excessive protein intake.

Calcium

Collection tube: red top
Normal values:
    Total: 8.8–10.0 mg/dL
    Ionized: 4.4–5.4 mg/dL

A calcium test measures the concentration of total calcium in the blood. It is used to evaluate parathyroid function, calcium metabolism, and malignancies.

Cholesterol

Collection tube: red top
Normal values: 140–220 mg/dL

Cholesterol testing is primarily used to detect disorders of blood lipids and to evaluate the risk potential for **atherosclerosis**, a disease in which arteries are narrowed by lipid deposits on the inner walls.

Chromosome Analysis

Specimen types: Leukocytes from peripheral blood collected in sodium heparin tube, bone marrow biopsies, fibroblasts from skin or surgical specimens, amniotic fluid, chorionic villus sampling, fetal tissue, or products of conception.

The test can be helpful in evaluation of several clinical situations. Some situations may be multiple malformations, failure to thrive, mental retardation, recurrent miscarriages, infertility, and delayed puberty. In addition, prenatal diagnosis of abnormalities may be detected, and certain cancers and leukemias may have the prognosis and/or stage of the disease determined.

Complete Blood Count (CBC)

Collection tube: lavender top
Normal values:
White blood cells (WBC): 4.5–11.0 thousand/mm^3
Red blood cells (RBC):
    Female: 4.2–5.4 million/mm^3
    Male: 4.6–6.2 million/mm^3
Hemoglobin (Hgb):
    Female: 12.6–15.8 g
    Male: 13.5–18.5 g
Hematocrit (Hct):
    Female: 36–47%
    Male: 40–54%
Mean corpuscular volume (MCV): 82–98 µl
Mean corpuscular hemoglobin (MCH): 27–31 picograms
Mean corpuscular hemoglobin concentration (MCHC): 32–36%

The CBC is used for basic screening in all patients. The phlebotomist will see it ordered frequently. The CBC gives information about the patient's diagnosis, prognosis, response to treatment, and recovery.

Cortisol

Collection tube: red top
Normal values:
    8:00 A.M.: 5–23 µg/dL
    4:00 P.M.: 3–15 µg/dL

A cortisol test is conducted to check adrenal hormone function.

Creatine Kinase (CK)

Collection tube: red top
Normal values:
    Male, 6–11 yr: 56–185 units/L
    Male, 12–18 yr: 35–185 units/L

Male, >19 yr: 38–174 units/L
Female, 6–7 yr: 50–145 units/L
Female, 8–14 yr: 35–145 units/L
Female, 15–18 yr: 20–100 units/L
Female, >19 yr: 96–140 units/L
Newborn: 68–580 units/L

Creatine kinase is an enzyme found in the heart and the skeletal muscles. The test is used to detect injury to myocardium and muscle. It is important in the diagnosis of myocardial infarction and skeletal muscle diseases such as muscular dystrophy. It may also detect central nervous system disorders such as Reye's syndrome.

CK can be divided into three isoenzymes: MM, BB, and MB. CK-MM is the isoenzyme that makes up almost all the circulatory enzymes in healthy persons. Skeletal muscle contains primarily CK-MM. Cardiac muscle contains both CK-MM and CK-MB. Brain tissue and the gastrointestinal and genitourinary tracts contain CK-BB. The isoenzyme studies help distinguish whether the CK originated from the heart (CK-MB) or the skeletal muscle (CK-MM).

Creatinine

Collection tube: red or green top
Normal values:
    Adult: 0.6–1.2 mg/dL
    Child: 0.3–0.7 mg/dL

A creatinine test is used to diagnose impaired renal (kidney) function.

Creatinine Clearance

24-hour urine collection and venous blood sample of 7 mL serum.

A blood and urine measurement that determines kidney function, primarily glomerular filtration. It measures the rate at which creatinine is cleared from the blood by the kidney.

Cytologic Study of Urine

Normal values:
    180 mL urine for adults
    10 mL urine for children

Urine cytology is useful in the diagnosis of cancer and inflammatory diseases of the bladder, the renal pelvis, the ureters, and the urethra.

The test is also valuable in detecting cytomegalic inclusion disease and other viral diseases. Urine should be as fresh as possible. If a delay is expected, an equal amount of 50% alcohol may be added as a preservative.

Digoxin

Collection tube: red top
Normal values:
  Therapeutic: 0.8–1.5 ng/mL
  Toxic: >25 ng/mL

Digoxin is a common heart medication. It is necessary to perform therapeutic drug monitoring to manage the individual patient's drug therapy.

Electrolytes (Sodium, Potassium, Chloride, CO_2 Content, Anion Gap)

Collection tube: red or green top
Normal values:
  Sodium: 134–148 mEq/L
  Potassium: 3.0–4.5 mEq/L
  Chloride: 100–112 mEq/L
  CO_2 content: 100–112 mEq/L
  Anion gap: 6–14 mEq/L

This panel of tests checks sodium, potassium, chloride, carbon dioxide, and anion gap substances in body fluids that are regulated by the lungs, kidneys, and glands.

Sodium is the electrolyte that offsets kidney activity for the discharge of toxins. Sodium is essential for the balance of bodily fluid levels. Organs involved with sodium function are the heart, kidneys, and adrenals. An elevated sodium level may be seen in kidney disorders, adrenal disorders, and intake of too little water. Decreased levels can be seen in liver, kidney, and heart disorders, adrenal and pituitary insufficiency, elevated blood sugar level, and intake of too much water.

Potassium is the mineral essential to heart and kidney function. It maintains heart rate, general muscle strength, normal nerve impulses, adrenal function, and the acid-base balance of the blood and urine. Increased levels can be seen in heart block, adrenal insufficiency, and hypoventilation. Decreased levels are seen in diarrhea, hyperadrenal conditions, general weakness, fatigue, irregular heartbeat, and chronic kidney disease.

Chloride is involved in adrenal, kidney, bladder, and bowel functions. Elevated levels are seen in kidney and adrenal disorders and bowel dysfunctions. Decreased levels can be seen in diarrhea, infection, diabetes, and hypoadrenalism.

Carbon dioxide content measures cellular toxic waste. It is vital to the acid-base balance and lung, kidney, and adrenal stability.

Anion gap reflects serum anion-cation balance and helps distinguish types of metabolic acidosis.

Ferritin

Collection tube: red top
Normal values:
    Men: 15–300 ng/mL
    Women: 12–150 ng/mL

Ferritin is the primary storage form that iron takes in the body.

Glucose (Random and Fasting)

Collection tube: green or red top
Normal values:
    Adult fasting: 70–110 mg/dL
    Fasting whole blood: 60–100 mg/dL
    Nonfasting: 80–125 mg/dL
    Child: 60–100 mg/dL

Glucose monitoring is used to detect any disorder of glucose metabolism and as an aid in diabetes management. In many cases, elevated blood sugar (hyperglycemia) indicates diabetes. In mild cases of diabetes, however, the blood sugar may be within normal ranges. In suspected cases of diabetes, a glucose tolerance test will be ordered (the patient consumes a sugared drink and then has blood drawn for up to six hours). A fasting blood sugar (FBS) level of > 140 mg/dL when confirmed by two or more tests is diagnostic of diabetes mellitus. In such a case, a glucose tolerance test should not be conducted. When glucose is < 30 mg/dL, brain damage is possible. When glucose is > 300 mg/dL, coma is possible.

Glucose (2-Hr Postprandial)

Collection tube: green or red top
Normal values: <120 mg/dL

The test sample is collected two hours after a meal, and is used as a screening test for diabetes.

Hemoglobin A1c

Collection tube: 5 mL lavender
Normal values: 6%–8% Alc

The glycosylated hemoglobin test is a diagnostic tool for monitoring diabetes therapy. The test is ordered every six to eight weeks and reflects diabetes control over several months.

HIV Antibody

Collection tube: red top
Normal values: nonreactive

This test is used to detect the presence of the antibody to the human immunodeficiency virus (HIV). It is used to screen blood and blood products. A positive result will be repeated and confirmed by Western blot or indirect fluorescent antibody testing.

Human Chorionic Gonadotropin (HCG)

Collection tube: red top, or urine sample
Normal values: negative in blood and urine

HCG levels are used to detect pregnancy in women or trophoblastic tumors in men. HCG can be detected in the urine of pregnant women 26 to 36 days after the first day of the last menstrual period, or 8 to 10 days after conception. Positive results may also occur with testicular tumors, and with cancer of the lung, stomach, colon, pancreas, or breast.

IgG and IgM

Collection tube: red top

Herpes simplex virus (HSV) is quite prevalent. It is often the most common cause of sexually transmitted disease. The test is used to determine the infectious status of pregnant patients in their last days of gestation. Testing for HSV antibody has also been used in bone marrow recipients and donors.

Iron

Collection tube: red top
Normal values:
    Transferrin: 240–480 mg/dL
    Total iron-binding capacity (TIBC): 240–450 mg/dL

Serum iron (men): 75–175 µg/dL
Serum iron (women): 65–165 µg/dL

Iron is a mineral essential for the formation of red blood cells and hemoglobin. It is also necessary for the function of the liver and spleen. Decreased iron levels can indicate iron deficiency, chronic diseases such as lupus, and physiologic stress such as from surgery or infection. Increased iron levels can indicate such problems as hemolytic anemias and acute hepatitis.

Lactic Acid Dehydrogenase (LD)

Collection tube: red top
Normal values: vary depending on direction of enzyme reaction and methodology used

The test is used to confirm myocardial or pulmonary infarction. It is also used as a tumor marker in seminoma or germ cell testis tumor.

Lipase

Collection tube: red top
Normal values: vary depending on methodology used

This test is used to diagnose pancreatitis.

Magnesium

Collection tube: red top
Normal values: 1.3–2.1 mEq/L

This test is used as an index of metabolic activity and for renal function. A reduced level can indicate renal failure, **cirrhosis** (inflammation) of the liver, alcoholism, and **colitis**, or inflammation of the colon.

Occult Blood in Stool

Tests for detecting blood in feces use substances that depend on peroxidase content as an indication of hemoglobin content to cause a color change in stool specimen. Feces should be collected in a dry, clean, urine-free container, or smeared onto a commercial prep kit. The normal person passes 2.0–2.5 mL of blood into the gastrointestinal tract daily. More than 2.8 mL of blood in a 24-hour period is a sign of disease. Detection of **occult** blood in the stool is very useful in detecting or localizing presence of blood in upper gastrointestinal bleeding. The test is especially important in screening for colonic carcinoma.

Osmolality

Collection tube: red top
Normal values: 275–295 m/osmol per kg

An osmolality test is used to assess fluid and electrolyte balance. Serum osmolality increases with dehydration and decreases with overhydration.

Ova and Parasites (O&P)

Warm stools are best for detecting ova and parasites. Do not refrigerate the specimen. A freshly passed stool is the best specimen. A stool the size of a walnut is adequate for testing. There are commercial collection kits that require that the specimen be divided and placed into separate vials.

The purpose of the test is to look for parasites and parasite eggs.
Stool Specimens for 24-, 48-, or 72-hour Collection.
All stools are collected for a period of 1, 2, or 3 days depending upon the physician's order.
The test is used with testing for fat and urobilinogen. The specimen should be placed in a one-gallon container from the laboratory. Save all stool. Keep refrigerated or place container in a cooler with canned ice.

Phenylketonuria (PKU)

Collection tube: none; a drop of blood is collected on filter paper
Normal values: <4 mg/100 mL

PKU is a genetic disease that can lead to mental retardation and brain damage if untreated. It can be detected in the blood of an affected child four days after birth, and in a child's urine two to eight weeks after birth.

Prothrombin Time (PT)

Collection tube: blue top
Normal values: 10–14 sec

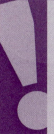

[**ALERT**]

Prothrombin Time is used as a screening test in diagnostic coagulation studies. It is ordered in conjunction with the management of anticoagulant therapy.

Renin

Collection tube: lavender top

Renin is an enzyme that converts angiotensinogen to angiotensin I. The test is most useful in the diagnosis of hypertension. In primary hyperaldosteronism, the findings will demonstrate that aldosterone secretion is exaggerated and secretion of renin is suppressed.

Rh Typing

Collection tube: red top
Normal values:
  Whites: 85% Rh-positive, 15% Rh-negative
  Blacks: 90% Rh-positive, 10% Rh-negative

Rh testing is done in conjunction with the ABO test. Human blood may be classified as Rh-positive or Rh-negative. The administration of Rh-positive blood to a recipient having Rh-negative blood could be fatal. In addition, Rh-negative pregnant women with Rh-positive partners may carry Rh-positive fetuses. In this case, cells from the fetus can pass through the placenta to the mother and cause production of antibodies in the maternal blood. The maternal antibodies can also pass through the placenta into the fetal blood and cause destruction of fetal blood cells. If this happens, reactions may range from anemia to death.

Rubella Antibody

Collection tube: red top
Normal values: <1.10 titer

Rubella testing is done to determine immune status and confirm rubella infection. A normal test result indicates that the patient is susceptible to the rubella virus. Higher values indicate the presence of the rubella antibody, and thus immunity or a current rubella infection.

Sedimentation Rate (Erythrocyte Sedimentation Rate, or ESR)

Collection tube: lavender top
Normal values:
  Westergren:
    Men: 0–15 mm/hr
    Women: 0–20 mm/hr

Wintrobe:
Men: 0–9 mm/hr
Women: 0–15 mm/hr

The ESR is the rate at which red cells settle out of unclotted blood in 1 hour. In inflammatory diseases, red cells become heavier and more likely to fall rapidly when placed in a special vertical test tube. The faster the cells settle, the higher the ESR. Sedimentation rate testing is often used to measure the progress of an inflammatory disease, rheumatic fever, rheumatoid arthritis, respiratory infections, and acute myocardial infarction. ESR is not considered diagnostic for any particular disorder.

Throat Culture

Specimen type: A sterile throat culture kit with polyester-tipped applicator or swab to swab the throat

Throat cultures are important in the diagnosis of streptococcal sore throat, diphtheria, thrush, tonsillar infection, gonococcal pharyngitis, and bordetella pertussis.

Triglycerides

Collection tube: lavender top
Normal values:
Men: 40–160 mg/dL (varies with age and diet)
Women: 35–135 mg/dL (varies with age and diet)

This test is used to evaluate patients with possible atherosclerosis. It is used as an indication of the body's ability to metabolize fat.

Uric Acid

Collection tube: red top
Normal values:
Men: 3.5–7.2 mg/dL
Women: 2.6–6.9 mg/dL

Measurement of uric acid is often used in the evaluation of renal failure, gout, and leukemia.

Urinalysis

10 mL of urine

Urinalysis is the means of determining various properties of urine, including color, odor, turbidity, specific gravity, pH, glucose, ketones, blood, protein, bilirubin, **urobilinogen**, nitrate, leukocyte esterase, and any abnormal constituents.

Vitamin B$_{12}$

Collection tube: red top
Normal values: 160–600 picograms/mL

This test is used to diagnose anemia. It is also helpful in conditions marked by a high turnover of myeloid cells, such as leukemia.

SUMMARY

With experience, the phlebotomist will become familiar with most common laboratory tests and their requirements. If the phlebotomist has any doubt about a test, laboratories have quick reference guides available. The phlebotomist must always be sure about all requirements before drawing blood. These requirements could include correct timing, refrigeration, special vials, and so on.

REVIEW ACTIVITIES

1. _____ is a test required of all blood donors and all potential blood recipients.

2. Rh typing must be done because _____.

3. ____ is an enzyme that is produced by the pancreas, salivary glands, ____, and fallopian tubes.

4. The ANA test is used to diagnose _____.

5. Aldolase is a glycolytic enzyme that catalyzes the breakdown of _____.

6. Alkaline phosphatase is an _____ originating mainly in _____, _____, and liver.

7. Blood cultures are used to detect _____.

8. In newborns, critical levels of bilirubin require aggressive treatment to prevent _____.

9. A CBC sample is collected in a _____-top tube.

10. Digoxin is a common _____ medication.

11. Electrolytes testing measures include:

    a. _____

    b. _____

    c. _____

    d. _____

    e. _____

12. _____ is a mineral essential to heart and kidney function.

13. Elevated blood sugar indicates _____.

14. The HIV antibody test is used to detect the presence of the antibody to the _____ virus.

15. Iron is a mineral essential for the formation of _____ and _____.

16. _____ is a genetic disease that can lead to mental retardation and brain damage if left untreated.

17. The APTT is a screening test for _____ disorders.

18. A rubella antibody test sample is collected in a _____-top tube.

19. An osmolality test is used to assess _____.

20. A cortisol test is used to check _____ hormone function.

▪ DISCUSSION QUESTION

1. You are preparing to draw a CBC, a Vitamin B-12, and an Iron on an outpatient. What diagnosis might the ordering physician be considering? Give an example of test results that may allow for a conclusive diagnosis.

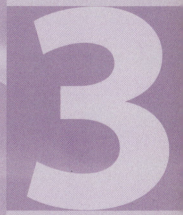

PART

3

Professional Success in Phlebotomy

11

Communication Skills for the Phlebotomist

"*Communication is not simply sending a message. It is creating true understanding—swiftly, clearly, and precisely.*"

—**Hitachi, Ltd.**

OBJECTIVES

After studying this unit, it is the responsibility of the learner to be able to:

1. Explain how speaking and communicating are different.
2. Give several examples of poor articulation.
3. List five types of nonverbal communication.
4. Describe the difference between hearing and listening.
5. Define the difference between listening and reflective listening.
6. Describe good telephone techniques.

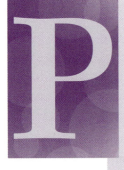

Phlebotomists interact with a large number of customers every day, including patients, physicians, coworkers, friends and family members of patients, and potential patients. One objective of each interaction should be to establish trust and rapport. Trust and rapport are partially the products of good communication. Research tells us that, on average, people spend 80 percent of their waking hours involved in some form of communication. That is why communication skills are as important for the phlebotomist as venipuncture and capillary puncture techniques.

Communication involves two active participants: the person sending a **message** and the person receiving the message. A message consists of whatever the sender communicates to the receiver. It is sent in the form of symbols, which can be either verbal or nonverbal. Verbal symbols are words. Nonverbal symbols include facial expressions, posture, appearance, tone of voice, and gestures. The receiver of the message is the listener, who must interpret the symbols.

■ THE SPEAKER

A common mistake we make as speakers is assuming that when we send a message, communication has taken place. Speaking and communication are not synonymous. We can speak to the listener, but if the message is not received in the manner in which it was meant to be understood, we have failed to communicate. For example, at one hospital's fitness clinic for persons recovering from heart attacks, a staff nurse gave a speech on cholesterol. "To decrease your cholesterol level," she said, "you should stop eating red meat." A few months later, she checked the cholesterol levels of the participants and discovered that one man's cholesterol level had risen slightly. "Did you stop eating red meat?" she asked. "Yes," he said. "I used to eat my steaks medium rare, but now I cook them until they are brown through and through." Communication had failed to take place between the nurse and the participant because the listener interpreted the message incorrectly. As speakers, we are responsible for sending messages that are understood by listeners. We can ensure this by using the appropriate words.

Appropriate Words

Occasionally in the medical profession, we are guilty of trying to impress our patients with our knowledge and skills. We do this by using terminology that is meant to impress, not express. Terms that are very common to the phlebotomist—such as *hematoma, CBC,* and *hemolysis*—are confusing to many patients. When trying to choose appropriate words, it is important to know something about the person or persons to whom you are speaking. There is no problem with using the word *hematoma* when speaking with fellow medical personnel. However, patients may be frightened if you tell them that a hematoma has formed and they do not know what that means.

Your goal should be to choose not the most sophisticated word, but the right word for the right person. Strive to build rapport with your patients by using words appropriate for their age and sex. If you are speaking to a 75-year-old patient, for example, stay away from slang that might not be understood. In fact, popular slang in general is not appropriate in the health care environment.

Use concrete and precise words. If your supervisor asks you for information about the day's workload, do not say, "It was really busy today." *Busy* is an abstract term that has different meanings for different people. Perhaps the supervisor thinks that busy means you performed 50 venipunctures by yourself that day, while you actually performed 30. Use concrete words to help you create the mental images that you want to convey. Instead of "It was really busy today," say "I performed 25 venipunctures this morning between six and nine." If the supervisor asks, "How did you do?" do not reply with something vague like, "They said I did a really good job." Who are "they," and what was the "really good job"? Be precise. Say, "The patients complimented me on my efficient, painless venipunctures."

Be brief and concise when giving information. If a patient should ask you why you are collecting a particular blood sample, say, "Your physician ordered a lab test." If the patient is persistent, simply say, "It would be best for you to have your physician explain it to you."

Articulation

Closely connected to choosing the appropriate word is choosing the appropriate manner in which to deliver the words. Your carefully chosen words deserve attention, to ensure clarity of delivery. Many of us are lazy in our daily conversations. We slur, mumble, drop syllables, and end up delivering poorly articulated messages. Look at the following conversation, for instance:

"Watcha doin?"

"Gettin ready to get an ASAP."

"Howbout that lass test? Wajagit?"

"Gotta red top."

"Can't ya useit?"

"Nah."

While poor **articulation** may not hurt us in conversation with our friends, it can hinder our communication with our patients. Enunciate words crisply and precisely.

Nonverbal Communication

Your personal appearance plays an important part in your communication. Your patients will start forming opinions about you before you open your mouth. You should always be clean, well groomed, and attractively dressed. Your attire should always be appropriate. Don't wear anything that would distract or offend your patients.

Establish immediate eye contact. Making good eye contact is important for three reasons:

- It demonstrates sincerity and interest.
- It creates a bond of communication and rapport between you and the patient.
- It enables you to get feedback from the patient. You can tell immediately if you have confused, angered, or pleased your patient.

If you are assisting a patient and another is waiting, acknowledge the waiting patient with brief eye contact and a smile. Do not ignore the patient. Patients deserve and appreciate being acknowledged.

Be aware of your posture. Good posture gives the impression of confidence and competence. Slouching projects inadequacy and disinterest. Do not lean against a bed, wall, or counter. Your patient will think you are too tired to perform your duties in a competent manner.

Smile sincerely at the patient. A warm smile will convey the message that you are pleased to see the patient and eager to provide a service. A sincere smile will put both you and your patient at ease.

A strong, clear voice will help you assert yourself and convey confidence. Research shows that if your tone of voice contradicts your words, patients will take the tone and inflection of your voice as the truth, rather than your words. In fact, 38 percent of your message *is* the tone of your voice. You should speak loudly enough for patients to understand you, but not so loudly that those not involved in your interaction will hear you.

Make sure your gestures are consistent with your verbal message. You convey a great deal with your body movements when you are communicating. Drumming your fingers on a table, crossing your arms, rolling your eyes upward, glancing at your watch, frowning, and casting your eyes down are just a few examples of negative nonverbal messages. In general, the key to an effective use of gestures is to avoid motions that may distract listeners from the message you wish to send.

■ THE LISTENER

Listening is another aspect of successful communication. Listening is following the thoughts of the speaker and understanding those thoughts as they were intended.

As a phlebotomist, you must be ready to listen at all times. Listening skills are not easily achieved. Many outside influences may interfere with your ability to listen effectively, and you may become distracted.

Conveying a message by speaking takes much longer than it takes to listen to the words. The average person speaks at the rate of 100 to 200 words per minute. However, a person can listen at a rate of 800 words per minute. During your "spare" time while listening, you might find yourself rehearsing what you are going to say to the patient, thinking about an argument with a coworker, or worrying about a dentist appointment that's coming up. But what you should be doing is focusing on what the speaker is saying.

According to Dr. Lyman Steil of the University of Minnesota,

> *"Tests have shown that immediately after listening to a ten-minute oral presentation, the average listener has heard, understood, properly evaluated, and retained approximately half of what was said. And within 48 hours, that drops off another 50 percent to a final 25 percent level of effectiveness. In other words, we quite often comprehend and retain only one quarter of what is said."*

Because we are patient-conscious phlebotomists, we not only want to listen to our patients, but we also want to listen reflectively. Listening reflectively means listening to the messages communicated by our patients and also letting them know that they are being heard and understood.

Reflective Listening

Reflective listening requires you to respond to a message while focusing on the speaker's need or problem. It involves two things:

1. Hearing and understanding through words and body language, and
2. Reflecting back what you have heard and seen.

There is a big difference between *hearing* and *listening*. When we hear, we experience sound waves vibrating on our eardrums. When we listen, we understand the words and take action accordingly. Many of us pretend to listen at times. Do not make this mistake with a patient. Patients are sensitive to facial cues such as a blank expression, unblinking eyes, or a faraway look. You may miss valuable information as well as send a message of disinterest. Additionally:

- Do not allow distractions to prevent listening. Do not focus your attention on the child crying in the next room or the sun shining through the window. Watch the speaker's face and take mental notes on the message. Do not form mental arguments with the patient. Do not prejudge.
- Ask questions. Make sure you have enough information.
- Acknowledge that you understand. Nod your head and say, "I understand."
- Summarize—reflect—what you heard. Take into account both the words and the nonverbal language. If the patient is quiet but has a frown, a flushed face, and a clenched jaw, you can say that you are observing anger. Repeat back the verbal message, using your own words.

■ TELEPHONE TECHNIQUES

Communicating on the telephone can be more difficult than communicating in person. We have to depend on fewer means for transmitting our message. Our customer cannot see our smiling face or our correct posture. We must rely on other factors to indicate our patient-conscious attitude.

PROCEDURE   Communicating on the Telephone

1. Answer each call by the third ring. If the phone is allowed to ring longer, the patient may already be irritated by the time you do answer.
2. Make your greeting brief, and use a pleasant tone of voice. State the name of your employer and your name. Example: "Sunny Oaks Medical Center Laboratory. This is Jackie. How may I help you?"

3. Answer multiple calls promptly; do not wait until you have finished with the first caller. Acknowledge the additional calls. Example: "Thank you for your patience. Would you please hold for just a moment?" If you suspect the first call may be lengthy, explain to the additional callers that you will be happy to return their call, and give them an idea of when you will do so.

4. Always acknowledge a ringing phone. A patient you are working with will hear the phone and prefer that you answer it to stop the ringing. Apologize to the patient who is with you and excuse yourself. Ask the caller to hold, or offer to return the call. Return as soon as possible to your original patient.

5. Transfer calls without making the caller angry. Make sure the caller has to state his request only to the first person who answers the telephone. If the patient has to repeat his request, he may become angry. Tell the caller that you are sorry but you need to transfer him to a person better able to help him. Give the caller the correct extension number for future reference; patients always appreciate being informed. When you transfer the call, give the pertinent information to the person answering the telephone.

6. Take complete telephone messages. Include the name of caller (ask for the correct spelling), the message, the date and time of day, and your name or initials.

7. Keep paper and a pen close to the telephone. Do not make the caller wait for you to find supplies.

8. Use the caller's name whenever possible. This may be the most effective way to establish rapport over the telephone.

9. Convey a professional manner. Do not chew gum or eat while answering the telephone. Keep the background noise to a minimum.

10. Use good communication techniques, such as a pleasant tone of voice, appropriate words, and clear enunciation.

■ SUMMARY

If you are not communicating well with a patient, even the best venipuncture technique possible may not result in a positive experience for your patient. Good communication skills are as important as excellent blood-drawing skills.

Phlebotomists must learn to use good speaking and listening skills. Choosing appropriate words, articulating properly, and projecting positive nonverbal messages are important skills for the phlebotomist. Listening carefully to the patient can make the difference between a bad experience and a positive one. Speaking and listening well on the telephone are very important as well.

■ REVIEW ACTIVITIES

1. The difference between speaking and communicating is:

   _____

   _____.

2. Give an example of a poorly articulated sentence and how it should be articulated properly.

   _____

   _____.

3. List five types of nonverbal communication.

   a. _____

   b. _____

   c. _____

   d. _____

   e. _____

4. Reflective listening is different from simple listening in that

   _____

   _____.

5. The steps taken by a person taking a telephone message should always include:

   a. _____

   b. _____

   c. _____

   d. _____

6. Describe the steps involved in handling multiple telephone calls.

   a. _____

   b. _____

   c. _____

◼ DISCUSSION QUESTIONS

1. You answer the telephone. The caller is obviously irate about something. He speaks rapidly and has a heavy accent that you have difficulty understanding. You think that possibly he wants information about a bill. How would you handle his call?

2. You have a coworker who accuses you of "not listening." Your supervisor talks with you about errors you have made in taking verbal instructions. What can you do to improve the situation?

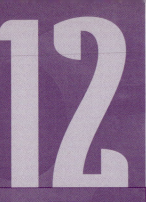

12

Conflict Management Skills

OBJECTIVES

After studying this unit, it is the responsibility of the learner to be able to:

1. Discuss the concept that conflict is natural and is not a win-or-lose situation.
2. Describe the five conflict management styles.
3. Determine and describe the learner's own conflict management style.
4. List the steps in conflict reduction.
5. List the steps in problem solving.
6. Apply conflict management skills to daily conflict situations.

"Conflict is natural; neither positive nor negative, it just is."

—Thomas F. Crum

KEY TERMS

accommodator one who aids, assists

avoider one who shuns, bypasses, evades

collaborator one who assists, acts as a partner

compromiser one who adapts, adjusts, negotiates

conflict clash, confrontation, difference, opposition, unrest

controller one who rules, manages

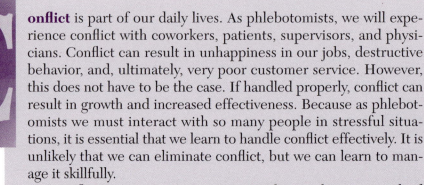

Conflict is part of our daily lives. As phlebotomists, we will experience conflict with coworkers, patients, supervisors, and physicians. Conflict can result in unhappiness in our jobs, destructive behavior, and, ultimately, very poor customer service. However, this does not have to be the case. If handled properly, conflict can result in growth and increased effectiveness. Because as phlebotomists we must interact with so many people in stressful situations, it is essential that we learn to handle conflict effectively. It is unlikely that we can eliminate conflict, but we can learn to manage it skillfully.

Conflict management is a process. When we become involved in a conflict, we must diagnose it and begin to take appropriate action to control the emotionality of the situation and enable the involved parties to understand and control their differences. We must understand that resolving a conflict is usually not about deciding who is right. It is about acknowledging and appreciating differences.

■ CONFLICT STYLES

We each have our own characteristic approach to handling conflict. While we experience many types of conflict—with a nurse upset about how long it took to have a glucose sample collected, a coworker unwilling to help with the workload, or a client refusing to have a blood specimen drawn, for example—we tend to respond in a consistent way. Our style is dependent on our past experiences and training. For instance, some people will try to avoid conflict at all costs. Others may be so concerned about "winning" that they must try to achieve their goals even at the risk of damaging or destroying their relationship with the other party. Joyce and William Wilmot describe the different approaches we take to conflict in their book, *Interpersonal Conflict.* They identify the following styles.

Collaborator

The **collaborator's** approach to conflict is to manage it by maintaining interpersonal relationships and ensuring that both parties to the conflict achieve their personal goals. The collaborator acts not only on behalf of his own interests, but also on behalf of the opposing party's interests. On recognizing that a conflict exists, the collaborator uses appropriate conflict management methods to solve the problem. This brings about a positive outcome for both parties. The underlying causes of the conflict are identified, and, through understanding, a solution is worked out. A problem-solving approach is used.

Compromiser

The **compromiser** assumes that all parties involved in the conflict cannot have completely positive outcomes. Compromisers bargain with respect to both the goals and the relationships of the involved parties, with persuasion and manipulation being the dominant approaches. The objective is to find some compromise that is mutually acceptable and that partially satisfies all parties involved.

Accommodator

The **accommodator's** approach to conflict involves maintaining the interpersonal relationship at all costs. The accommodator has little or no concern for identifying and understanding the source of the conflict. Giving in, appeasing, and avoiding conflict are viewed as ways of protecting the relationship. The conflict is smoothed over in an attempt to make everything "OK." The accommodator's role is that of peacemaker.

Controller

The **controller** tries to overpower the opposing party in an authoritarian manner, whatever the cost to the relationship involved. Conflict is viewed as a win-or-lose proposition. Finger pointing is more important than identifying the source of the conflict. A culprit must be identified and punished. This is a power-oriented mode; the controller uses whatever power is appropriate and available to achieve the desired resolution.

Avoider

The **avoider's** approach is to view conflict as something to be ignored or avoided. Controversy or disagreement is viewed as unhealthy. A central theme in this style is hopelessness, which results in a high degree of frustration for all parties involved. Personal goals are usually not met, nor is the interpersonal relationship maintained in this style of conflict. Avoiding conflict might take the form of diplomatically diverting an issue, postponing dealing with an issue until a better time, or simply withdrawing from a threatening situation. Avoiders "absorb" until they become so unhappy that they react inappropriately to a situation.

■ CONFLICT MANAGEMENT

A common situation involving conflict is the distribution of a department's workload. Phlebotomists often complain that they "do more" than their coworkers, and that they have to do "harder sticks." When the morning's assignments are distributed, for instance, how might the collaborators, compromisers, accommodators, controllers, or avoiders in your department handle the workload?

The following survey asks questions about situations that you are likely to encounter in your personal and professional life. After reading about each situation and the five possible responses, circle the letter for the response that would be most typical for you. Use other work-related conflicts you have experienced as your frame of reference, and keep those situations in mind when responding to the survey. (There are no right or wrong responses.)

1. On experiencing strong feelings in a disagreement with a coworker concerning who will obtain blood samples from an unpleasant and combative client, you

   a. enjoy the emotional release and sense of exhilaration and accomplishment.

   b. enjoy the strategizing involved and the challenge of the conflict.

   c. think seriously about how others are feeling.

   d. find it frightening, because you do not accept that differences can be discussed without hurting. You begrudgingly collect the specimens.

   e. become convinced that there is nothing you can do to resolve the issue.

2. What do you believe are the best results that can come out of conflict?

   a. Conflict helps people face the fact that one answer is better than others.

   b. Conflict results in canceling out extremes of thinking so that a strong middle ground can be reached.

   c. Conflict clears the air and enhances commitment and results.

   d. Conflict demonstrates the absurdity of self-centeredness and draws people closer together in their commitment to each other.

   e. Conflict lessens complacency and assigns blame where it belongs.

3. When you become angry with a coworker, you

   a. verbally attack and "get it off your chest."

   b. try to smooth things over with a good story.

   c. express your anger in a respectful manner and invite your coworker to respond.

    d. try to compensate for your anger by acting in a way opposite to what you are feeling.

    e. remove yourself from the situation.

4. When you find yourself disagreeing with other members of a group on an important issue, you

    a. defend your position.

    b. appeal to the logic of the group in the hope of convincing at least a majority that you are right.

    c. explore points of agreement and disagreement and the feelings of the group's members, and then search for alternatives that take everyone's views into account.

    d. go along with the rest of the group.

    e. do not participate in the discussion and do not feel bound by any decision reached.

5. When you see the conflict emerging in a group, you

    a. push for any quick decision, to ensure that the task is completed or a resolution is reached.

    b. avoid outright confrontation by moving the discussion toward a middle ground, without identifying the real nature of the conflict.

    c. share with the group your impression of what is going on, so that the nature of the impending conflict can be discussed.

    d. forestall or divert the conflict before it emerges by distracting the involved parties with humor.

    e. stay out of the conflict.

Scoring the Survey

This survey is not intended as an absolute method for determining your style of conflict management. Rather, it is a means of helping you to expand your awareness of how you typically respond to conflict. It is not unusual to respond to conflicts with a combination of styles, depending on the circumstances of each situation. You may determine your predominant style by totaling the number of responses under each answer category. The most frequently circled letter reflects your conflict management style:

    a. controller

    b. compromiser

    c. collaborator

    d. accommodator

    e. avoider

■ PROBLEM SOLVING

Managing conflict to achieve a positive resolution requires conflict reduction and problem solving. In conflict reduction, the emotionality of the situation is reduced. The actual problem-solving work comes next. To arrive at a positive resolution, the following things must be done:

- The problem must be seen as external to the involved parties. It must be a "we" problem rather than a "me" problem; no finger pointing is allowed.
- The parties must describe the problem in terms of their similar needs and interests.
- The emphasis must be on goals or benefits that can be achieved with a solution that is not predetermined by one or both parties.
- The conflict must be focused on facts and issues, not personalities.
- The emphasis must be placed on long-term effects, not just the immediate disagreement.

Steps to Conflict Reduction

1. Listen to the other party's position. Develop rapport by sincerely trying to understand that position. Summarize for the other party what you have heard.
2. Clearly state your position, and explain why you feel the way you do.
3. Ask the other person or persons to explain why they feel as they do.
4. Summarize and come to an agreement on what your differences really are.
5. Move on to problem solving.

Steps to Problem Solving

1. Define the problem in a nonthreatening way. Do not place blame.
2. Identify all possible solutions. Do not evaluate.
3. Evaluate options that are satisfactory to both parties.
4. Decide on an acceptable solution.
5. Decide how to implement the solution.
6. Develop a process for evaluating the success of the solution.

■ SUMMARY

By properly managing conflict, we can take a stressful situation, such as conflict over how work is distributed, and use it to develop more positive, productive relationships. Phlebotomists should make the conflict management process a routine part of their job. Individual phlebotomists, as well as their departments, can benefit from conflict if they remember that conflict is natural. It is what you do with the conflict that makes a difference.

■ REVIEW ACTIVITIES

1. The collaborator's approach to conflict is to:

_____

_____

2. The compromiser's approach to conflict is to:

_____

_____

3. The accommodator's approach to conflict is to:

_____

_____

4. The controller's approach to conflict is to:

_____

_____

5. The avoider's approach to conflict is to:

_____

_____

■ DISCUSSION QUESTIONS

1. What is your conflict management style? How can you make adjustments to your style to make a conflict a positive experience?

2. Think of a situation when a conflict in which you were involved ended in a very unproductive manner. What could you have done differently?

13

Becoming a Professional

OBJECTIVES

After studying this unit, it is the responsibility of the learner to be able to:

1. Name five qualities an employer desires in an employee.
2. Describe three ways to demonstrate loyalty to an employer, coworkers, and a supervisor.
3. List three ways to demonstrate reliability.
4. Discuss three ways that teamwork may be demonstrated.
5. Describe how a willingness to accept change may be demonstrated.
6. List several ways pride in the performance of job duties may be shown.
7. Summarize the personnel policies regarding a drug-free workplace, violence-free workplace, sexual harassment, and worker's compensation.
8. List six different external customers with whom the phlebotomist will interact.
9. List four different internal customers with whom the phlebotomist will interact.
10. State six questions phlebotomists can ask themselves that will indicate their own level of customer service motivation.
11. List 10 qualities that customers want from their service provider.
12. Give 10 examples of how phlebotomists can respond to the 10 qualities desired by customers.

KEY TERMS

access availability

communication the transmission of information

competence proficiency, skill, knowledge

courtesy respect, consideration, attention, manners, politeness

credibility integrity, trustworthiness, honesty

customer anyone to whom a service or a product is provided

external customer someone to whom a service is provided who is not employed by the health care facility

internal customer someone to whom a service is provided who is an employee of the health care facility

loyalty firm allegiance

reliability accurate, dependable performance

responsiveness readiness to provide prompt service

security assurance, certainty, safety

tangibles things that are actual and concrete

teamwork the subordination of the individual's tasks or goals to the common purpose of the group

understanding appreciation, sensitivity, comprehension

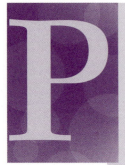

Phlebotomists will interact with many different types of **customers**—persons to whom they provide a service. Most customers will be pleasant, rational people. Some will be difficult, eccentric, or irrational. Regardless, the phlebotomist must provide all customers with efficient, top-quality service that conveys a caring attitude and a willingness to please. It is this type of service that will create satisfied, returning customers. This chapter will focus on delivering those services in a customer-oriented manner.

HEALTH CARE CUSTOMERS

Phlebotomists are the laboratory's most visible customer service staff. They supply their services to a variety of customers, both external and internal. The most obvious **external customer** is the patient. Patients are the reason phlebotomists come to work every day. Physicians are also external customers. Other external customers include physicians' office staff, other health care facilities, third-party payers, and different organizations in the community. **Internal customers** are nurses, pathologists, other departments within the laboratory, and all other departments within the hospital to whom the phlebotomists provide a service. All of these customers want a different service. And they all prefer that those services be delivered in a customer-oriented manner.

CUSTOMER SATISFACTION

Phlebotomists should understand that serving customers is their primary function. They serve the customer by collecting laboratory specimens. A satisfied customer may be the most important reward received at the end of a day's work. Phlebotomists should ask themselves daily:

- Do I believe in my employer, its service, and the service I am giving?
- Do I listen to customers who have a problem, a question, or a special request? Or am I too eager to say, "That's not in my job description"?
- Do I take action to solve problems, answer questions, and handle special requests?

- Do I accept the responsibility for any inconvenience or misunderstanding caused by my organization?
- Do I do everything within my power to satisfy the needs of every customer?
- Do I recommend service enhancement ideas to my supervisor?

The phlebotomist should be able to answer "yes" to each of these questions.

Customer satisfaction plays a very important role in the success of a business. Research done by Texas A & M University found that customers are looking for these qualities:

- **Reliability:** accurate, dependable performance
- **Responsiveness:** readiness to provide prompt service
- **Tangibles:** proper appearance of the facility, equipment, and personnel
- **Competence:** possession of requisite skills and knowledge
- **Courtesy:** politeness, respect, consideration, and friendliness
- **Communication:** willingness to keep customers informed
- **Credibility:** trustworthiness, believability, and honesty
- **Security:** freedom from danger, risk, or doubt
- **Understanding:** knowledge of customers; willingness to learn customer requirements and provide personal attention
- **Access:** convenient hours and location; ease of contact

Professional phlebotomists may demonstrate each of the customer service requirements in the following ways.

Reliability

Collect blood samples using appropriate, accurate procedures, not taking shortcuts. Answer questions in a knowledgeable manner. Refer difficult questions to the appropriate person. Identify patients, collect the samples in the correct collection tubes, and handle and transport specimens in the proper manner.

Responsiveness

Collect urgent, timed, and as-soon-as-possible specimens within appropriate time frames. Answer the telephone within three rings. Take care of problems without "passing the buck." Accept assignments promptly and graciously. Answer questions and requests for help in a timely manner.

Tangibles

Keep your work area clean and neat. Maintain a well-groomed and professional appearance. Keep a neat and well-organized collection tray.

Competence

Stay up-to-date on new procedures and policies. Attend staff meetings and educational in-service workshops. Expand your knowledge by reading material pertaining to the phlebotomy field.

Courtesy

Say "please" and "thank you." Introduce yourself to patients and new coworkers. Help coworkers when your assignment is finished. Compliment others on a job well done. Greet people with a smile. Do not vent anger and frustrations on patients and coworkers. Do not blame others for your mistakes. Explain procedures to patients before beginning them. Be aware of your nonverbal behavior, and strive to make it consistent with positive behavior. Treat people the way you would like to be treated. Do not spread rumors or support negative behavior.

Communication

Keep the supervisor informed of problems and potential problems. Keep coworkers informed of special situations. Be open and honest about feelings rather than talking about someone behind their back.

Credibility

Admit mistakes. Tell the truth.

Security

Make patients feel comfortable and secure. Demonstrate confidence in your skills.

Understanding and Knowing the Customer

Call patients by name (Mr., Mrs., Ms. Jones). Remember returning patients' special interests. Remember special requests from patients.

Phlebotomists are very fortunate to be able to represent their employer in a frontline role. Most laboratory employees rarely have the opportunity to interact with so many different customers. To succeed in this job, the phlebotomist must enjoy working with and helping people. Customers expect quality service. They also expect service to be provided in a considerate and respectful manner. Phlebotomists must continually reflect an attitude that says, "We are professionals, and we care about you as our customer." Customer satisfaction is built on positive communication and concern, and on the human relationships that exist between those being served and those providing the service.

PREPARING FOR PROFESSIONALISM

Taking the national phlebotomy certification exam should be the first priority of the student immediately after completing the phlebotomy courses. There are several organizations available that offer certification exams for phlebotomists. However, take time to research the best choice for you. Select the certifying agency that is best for you. Make phone calls to your local hospitals, clinics, etc., to see which certification they prefer. If you plan to move to a new location in another state, call health care facilities in the city where you plan to live. Some certifying organizations are not reputable or not in good standing with the Better Business Bureau.

PHLEBOTOMY CERTIFICATION

Phlebotomist-Certifying Agencies

ACA

American Certification Agency
P.O. Box 58
Osceola, IN 46561
www.acacert.com
Phone: (574) 277-4538

AMT

American Medical Technologists
710 Higgins Road
Park Ridge, IL 60068-5765
http://www.amt1.com
Phone: (847) 823-5169 or (800) 275-1268

ASCP

American Society of Clinical Pathologists
2100 West Harrison Street
Chicago, IL 60612-3798

http:www.ascp.org/
Phone: (312) 738-1336

NCA

National Credentialing Agency
PO Box 15945-289
Lenexa, KS 66285
www.nca-info.org
Phone: (913) 599-5340

■ RESEARCHING POTENTIAL EMPLOYMENT

Beginning a Job Search

The best time to begin a job search is when you begin your phlebotomy courses. The current job market is very competitive, and you need to take every opportunity to place yourself ahead of your competitors. Successfully completing your internship is the first step to becoming employed. While working as an intern, take time to network with staff in your department as well as in other departments. Establish a reputation of reliability, helpfulness, and honesty. Be on time, show enthusiasm by asking good questions, and offer to help whenever possible. Be a team player, don't contribute to gossip, and learn to enjoy everyone's company. Don't become part of a clique. Look professional every day. Take time to look your best as if you were interviewing for a job opening. Make an effort to express your thanks to the supervisor and staff for investing their time and knowledge in your future. When your internship is completed, ask to meet with the supervisor briefly. Make your interest in employment known, and leave your resume with current phone number and address.

Utilizing the Internet

The Internet offers vast opportunities in helping you with your job search. Tips for writing a resume, interviewing, and follow-up methods are often free. In addition, the Internet provides you with an opportunity to search job postings without leaving your home. You save time and car expenses while searching in the comfort of your home. When you do find job openings that interest you, start an organized method of documenting your job applications. You can create a spreadsheet on your computer, or perhaps use an index card system to record the date and potential employer. Review your records frequently so that you are not applying multiple times to the same job posting. You can also use the system to help you make follow-up calls.

The Interview

Make certain that you have correct information concerning the time of your interview, where the interview will take place, and with whom the interview is scheduled. Arrive shortly ahead of time. Arriving several minutes ahead of the scheduled time is inconvenient to the interviewer. You may interrupt an interview with another applicant, or you may interrupt other job requirements of the interviewer. Arriving late is definitely bad etiquette. Leave your home early enough so that you can allow for any unexpected event. Dress appropriately for the job position. Take time to come to the health care facility before you come for the interview. Notice how the staff dresses. Use your observations as a guide for selecting your dress. Overdressing makes a negative impression just as underdressing does. If you need a haircut, get one! If your shoes need polishing, polish them! Don't use overpowering perfume or cologne. If you smoke, don't smoke just prior to the interview. The smell of cigarette smoke may be offensive to the interviewer. When you greet the interviewer, establish eye contact. Speak with confidence, and smile occasionally. A smile goes a long way to establish rapport with the interviewer. Tell the truth and do not exaggerate. Do not offer negative information. Do not speak negatively of previous employers. Ask good questions. Always thank the interviewer for their time, and shake their hand.

Follow-Up

Appropriate follow-up may get you the job. The interviewer is probably very busy. Do not take up too much of their time. Make your phone call brief and pleasant. Ask when a decision will be made. Thank the interviewer for their time, and let them know that you are very interested in working at their facility. Do not make any further calls to the interviewer. Wait for a job offer, and if it does not come, move on to other possibilities.

Keep Looking

While you are waiting for a decision concerning your interview, keep up the job search. Don't just confine you search to your "dream" job. Look for opportunities within a health care facility for which you may be qualified. Taking a clerical position is worthy of your time while you wait for a phlebotomy position to be come available. There are several job possibilities in various departments that would be interested in hiring someone with your educational experience. Apply for as many job openings as you possibly can.

There are many qualities that employers appreciate in an employee. It is not possible to discuss all of those qualities here. However, this chapter will focus on five qualities that are extremely important.

QUALITIES OF THE SUCCESSFUL EMPLOYEE

Loyalty

Loyalty is a quality employers expect of any employee. If you do not believe in your employer and the goals and philosophy of the organization, you are doing yourself and your employer a great disservice. Being loyal to your employer includes being loyal to your supervisor, coworkers, and patients. Loyalty does not mean agreeing with every idea or concept that comes from management. However, loyalty does mean handling disagreements in the proper manner. These are some guidelines for demonstrating loyalty:

- Do not complain about concerns to someone who is powerless to change the situation.
- Do not complain about work problems to patients.
- Take concerns to your immediate supervisor and present them in a positive manner by offering solutions.
- If your employer is unable or unwilling to change the situation that troubles you, you should support your organization's decision or find another employer. You do not have the option to create discord among coworkers by rallying support for your cause.
- Demonstrate a willingness to help an employer through difficult times. Be willing to work an occasional extra shift or overtime if there are staffing shortages. Be thrifty with supplies. Difficult times for an employer may mean difficult times ahead for you if you are unwilling to contribute to your employer's success.
- Demonstrate loyalty to coworkers by refusing to take part in gossip. Excuse yourself from such conversations, or offer a positive statement about the individual being discussed. Gossip can do a great deal of harm and is very difficult to control.

Elbert Hubbard, author, says this about loyalty:

> *"If you work for a man, in heaven's name, work for him. If he pays you wages which supply you bread and butter, work for him; speak well of him; stand by him and stand by the institution he represents. If put to a pinch, an ounce of loyalty is worth a pound of cleverness. If you must vilify, condemn, and eternally disparage—resign your position, and when you are outside, damn to your heart's content, but as long*

as you are part of the institution do not condemn it. If you do that, you are loosening the tendrils that are holding you to the institution, and at the first high wind that comes along, you will be uprooted and blown away, and probably will never know the reason why."

Reliability

Reliability means consistently doing what is expected of you. You may demonstrate your reliability in several ways:

- Maintain an acceptable attendance record. Make every effort to arrive at work on time, as scheduled. Do not call in sick when you are not ill. Plan vacation days ahead of time and give the dates to your supervisor well in advance.
- Complete assigned duties on time and in a high-quality manner. If unable to complete an assignment, notify the supervisor and ask for suggestions on how to proceed.
- Keep your word. If you have offered to help with a project, follow through.

Teamwork

Every duty that a phlebotomist performs involves **teamwork**. The team may consist of fellow phlebotomists, laboratory staff, or the entire health care organization. Here are some ways to play your part as an effective team member:

- Offer to help others when the workload allows.
- Offer positive criticism to a new coworker by suggesting how to perform tasks more efficiently or accurately.
- Do not take pleasure in finding mistakes made by others. The quality of your coworkers' work also reflects on you. You succeed when your coworkers succeed.
- Work to achieve the goals of the department and the organization.

Be Open to Change

Perhaps one of the most important qualities needed to work in the medical field is an openness to change. You can demonstrate that you are open to change in the following ways:

- Be flexible in scheduling. Your supervisor may need to try different and creative scheduling ideas to make the department as productive as possible. Your willingness to be flexible may prevent a reduction in staff.

- Be willing to be trained in new duties. Having multiple skills may be necessary in health care's current environment.
- Stay informed, and offer suggestions for improvement.
- Be willing to assist where needed. Ask for training if you feel inadequate in performing a duty.

Take Pride in Your Work

Employees who take **pride** in their work perform every duty to the best of their ability. You can perform at your very best in these ways:

- Take good care of yourself physically, mentally, and emotionally. Get enough sleep and exercise. Eat proper meals. If you are having personal problems, seek counseling or advice from a source that can help you. An unhappy employee is not a productive employee.
- Do not take shortcuts in performing your duties. Take time to do things right the first time.
- Look for ways to improve. Do not stagnate. Read about your profession. Attend in-service workshops. Set new goals when old goals are achieved.

Know Your Employer's Personnel Policies

It is important to know your employer's personnel policies so that you may act and perform in a manner acceptable to your institution. It is also important to know the policies so that you may understand your rights and protections.

Equal Employment Opportunity

The employer must comply with federal, state, and local laws governing Equal Employment Opportunity (EEO). The employer must provide equal opportunity to all employees and applicants so that no person shall incur unlawful discrimination in employment because of race, religion, color, sex, age, national origin, ancestry, disability, sexual orientation, and veteran status in matters of employment. It is strictly prohibited to discriminate unlawfully against any employee or applicant.

It is the responsibility of all members of management to follow this principle, and to ensure that employees under their supervision are familiar with and follow this principle. As an employee, the phlebotomist is responsible for becoming familiar with the EEO principles and supporting them. You are to report alleged violations to your supervisor or to a human resources representative. You will be provided confidentiality and will be protected from retaliation to the extent practicable.

Drug-Free Workplace

Most employers are dedicated to ensuring quality patient services. Employees are expected to perform their responsibilities unencumbered by the presence of drugs, narcotics, controlled substances, or alcohol. Prescribed drugs are acceptable when used in a manner intended unless job performance is affected. Employers may conduct drug and alcohol screening when management determines that reasonable suspicion exists to suggest that an employee is impaired, or is using or possessing a controlled substance or alcohol on the job. The screening process is conducted according to specific protocols at each institution. Employees found to be in violation of the drug-free policy are subject to discipline, including termination. Perhaps they may be required to complete a substance abuse rehabilitation program as a condition of continued employment.

Sexual Harassment

Sexual harassment is prohibited in any form, including verbal, physical, or visual harassment. Sexual harassment includes unwelcome sexual advances, requests for sexual favors, and other verbal or physical conduct of a gender-discriminatory nature in the following circumstances:

- Acceptance of the conduct is made either a term or condition of employment.
- Acceptance or rejection of the conduct is used as the basis for employment decisions affecting the employee.
- The conduct is intended for or has the effect of interfering with an individual's work performance or creates an intimidating, hostile, or offensive work environment.

A phlebotomist who feels he or she has been sexually harassed should contact a manager or human resources representative. The phlebotomist will be provided confidentiality and will be protected from retaliation to the extent practicable. A report and investigation will follow with appropriate action taken.

Violence-Free Workplace

Your employer is committed to maintaining a safe environment for patients, employees, physicians, visitors, and the public. Acts such as intimidation, threatening or hostile physical or verbal behaviors, stalking, physical or verbal abuse, assault, vandalism, arson, sabotage, possession or use of weapons, and jokes or offensive comments regarding violence will not be allowed. If the phlebotomist has felt subjected to or has observed any of these behaviors, it should be reported immediately to the manager, security department, or human resources representative.

Phlebotomists may also contact the local law enforcement authorities first if it is felt the situation is immediately dangerous to their own safety or that of others. The matter will be documented and investigated, and appropriate action will be taken.

Worker's Compensation

A phlebotomist who sustains a work-related injury or illness should notify the manager immediately. The employee is required by law to complete the Employee Incident Report within four working days of the incident. Failure to do so may result in a forfeit of compensation. The employer will designate care providers who will treat all work-related injuries and illnesses. Suspected exposures to communicable diseases should be reported immediately to the supervisor. Exposure to body fluids must be reported immediately to the supervisor. Lost work time will be paid compensation.

■ SUMMARY

Your success as a phlebotomist will depend on your own willingness to succeed in your job. You must be alert to growth opportunities, be properly prepared to take them, and accept them with enthusiasm.

■ REVIEW ACTIVITIES

1. A customer may be defined as _____.

2. _____ are the laboratory's most visible customer service staff.

3. Examples of the phlebotomist's external customers include:

   a. _____

   b. _____

   c. _____

   d. _____

   e. _____

4. Examples of the phlebotomist's internal customers include:

   a. _____

   b. _____

   c. _____

   d. _____

5. A phlebotomist may demonstrate reliability by:

   a. _____

   b. _____

   c. _____

6. Responsiveness may be demonstrated by:

   a. _____

   b. _____

   c. _____

   d. _____

   e. _____

7. Competence may be demonstrated or enhanced by:

   a. _____

   b. _____

   c. _____

   d. _____

   e. _____

8. Some ways in which courtesy may be expressed to the customer are:

   a. _____

   b. _____

   c. _____

   d. _____

   e. _____

   f. _____

9. A phlebotomist may demonstrate good communication skills by:

   a. _____

   b. _____

10. Demonstrating credibility means:

    a. _____

    b. _____

11. Making the patient feel comfortable is an example of providing

_____.

12. Calling patients by name and remembering their special interests is how _____ may be expressed to the patient.

13. Name five qualities that an employer desires in an employee.

    a. _____

    b. _____

    c. _____

    d. _____

    e. _____

14. Loyalty may be demonstrated by:

    a. _____

    b. _____

    c. _____

15. Reliability may be demonstrated by:

    a. _____

    b. _____

    c. _____

16. A specific example of working as part of a team would be

_____

_____

_____.

17. Phlebotomists may demonstrate pride in their work by:

    a. _____

    b. _____

    c. _____

    d. _____

18. A willingness to accept necessary change may be demonstrated by:

    a. _____

    b. _____

    c. _____

    d. _____

■ DISCUSSION QUESTIONS

1. You have a coworker who is constantly telling "dumb blonde" jokes, and calls the women staff "honey," "babe," and "sweetie." Your coworkers do not seem to mind, and laugh at his jokes. You, however, find his comments offensive. You do not want to alienate the group, and are afraid of telling him that you are offended. What should you do?

2. You find yourself being very short-tempered with a coworker over her unwillingness to repay a small loan of money. You ask your supervisor to talk to her, but the supervisor says it is not a work-related matter. You decide to pressure her into repaying the loan by telling all of your coworkers that she is a cheap jerk. You keep patient information from her that is needed to draw blood samples. What are the issues with this situation? How should it be handled?

3. You stick yourself with a contaminated needle. You do not want to report it because it is your third accidental stick. The department states that you must be drug-tested for your third incident. You are fearful of losing your job if you report the accident. What should you do? Why?

4. A patient arrives in the outpatient lab stating that she needs to have a blood test. She has not registered as a patient, she has no physician orders with her, and she is on her lunch break and must be back at work within an hour. She also says she had blood drawn a week earlier and complains that the phlebotomist "stuck her four times before getting a blood sample." What would you do?

5. An inpatient is upset when you arrive in his room to obtain a blood sample. He states that he has had his "call light" on for over 45 minutes. He needs assistance to get to the restroom. What would you do?

Student Name: _____

Procedure	Needs Improvement	Approved	Reviewed by	Date
Greet patient				
Identify patient				
Explain procedure				
Select venipuncture site				
Assemble equipment				
Put on gloves				
Tie tourniquet				
Prep puncture site				
Inspect needle for flaws				
Anchor vein				
Stretch skin taut				
Bevel up				
Needle properly anchored				
Puncture vein smoothly				
Collection tube inserted into holder				
Tube top punctured				
Specimens collected in proper order				
Tubes removed from holder.				
Invert tubes 4–5 times.				
Tourniquet released				
Bluntable needle activated				
Needle withdrawn from vein properly				
Pressure applied to venipuncture site with gauze				
Dispose of needle				
Bandage applied if appropriate				
Tubes labeled with required information				
Tubes bagged for transport				
Remove gloves				
Wash hands				
Thank patient				
Leave room environment as found				
Transport specimens to laboratory				

References

American Hospital Association. *The Patient Care Partnership*. www.aha.org.

Beauchamp, T., & Childress, J. (1989). *Principles of biomedical ethics.* New York: Oxford University Press.

Bendiner, E., & Bendiner, J. (1990). *Biographical dictionary of medicine.* New York: Facts On File, Inc.

Blake, R., & Moulton, J. (1964). *The managerial grid.* Houston: Gulf Publishing.

Centers for Disease Control and Prevention. *Isolation Guidelines*. www.cdc.gov/ncidod/ hiip/isolat/isopart2.htm.

Daigneault, R. (1990). A surprise visit from OSHA. *Medical Laboratory Observer,* (January), 31–34.

Daintith, J., & Isaacs, A. (1989). *Medical quotes.* Oxford, UK: Market House Books Ltd.

Davies, G. H., Davies, N. E., & Sanders, E. D. (1988). William Cobbett, Benjamin Rush, and the death of General Washington. *Journal of the American Medical Association,* (February), 912–915.

Fischbach, F. (1992). *Laboratory and diagnostic tests.* Philadelphia: J. B. Lippincott.

Gottfried, E. L., & Adachi, M. M. (1997). Prothrombin time and activated partial thromboplastin time can be performed on the first tube. *AM J Clin Pathol,* 107(6), 681–683.

Guthrie, D. (1946). *A history of medicine.* Philadelphia: J. B. Lippincott.

Haller, J. S. (1986). Decline of bloodletting: A study in 19th-century ratiocinations. *Southern Medical Journal,* (April), 469–475.

Holtke, L. B. (2006). *The complete textbook of phlebotomy.* Clifton Park, NY: Thomson Delmar Learning.

Jamieson, B., & Hurwitz, S. (1994, April). *Pediatric blood collections.* Denver: American Society of Clinical Pathologists Teleconference.

Katz, N. H., & Lawyer, J. W. (1985). *Communication and conflict resolution skills.* Dubuque, IA: Kendall/Hunt Publishing.

Lindh, W., Pooler, M. S., Tamparo, D. C., & Cerrato, J. U. (1994). *Comprehensive medical assisting, administrative and clinical competencies.* Clifton Park, NY: Thomson Delmar Learning.

McCord, C. P. (1970). Bloodletting and bandaging. *Archives of Environmental Health,* (April), 551–558.

McManus, J. F. A. (1963). *The fundamental ideas of medicine.* Springfield, IL: Charles C. Thomas.

National Committee for Clinical Laboratory Standards (NCCLS): Protection of Laboratory Workers from Occupationally Acquired Infections, Approved Guideline, 2nd ed. NCCLS Document M29-A. Wayne, PA: NCCLS, 2001.

National Committee for Clinical Laboratory Standards (NCCLS): Blood Collection on Filter Paper for Newborn Screening Programs, Approved Standard, 4th ed. NCCLS Document LA4-A4. Wayne, PA: NCCLS, July 2003.

National Committee for Clinical Laboratory Standards (NCCLS): Procedures for the Collection of Diagnostic Blood Specimens by Venipuncture, Approved Standard, 5th ed. NCCLS Document H3-A5. Wayne, PA: NCCLS, December 2003.

National Committee for Clinical Laboratory Standards (NCCLS): Tubes and Additives for Venous Blood Specimen Collection, Approved Standard, 5th ed. NCCLS Document H1-A5l. Wayne, PA: NCCLS, 2003.

National Committee for Clinical Laboratory Standards (NCCLS): Procedures and Devices for the Collection of Diagnostic Capillary Blood specimens, Approved Standard. NCCLS Document H4-A5. Wayne, PA: NCCLS, 2004.

Occupational Safety and Health Administration (OSHA): Revised Bloodborne Pathogens Standard 1910.1030. Needlestick Safety and Prevention Bill Act. April 18, 2001.

Occupational Safety and Health Administration (OSHA): Re-Use of Blood Tube Holders, Standard Interpretations. June 12, 2002, www.osha.gov.

Occupational Safety and Health Administration (OSHA): Re-Use of Blood Tube Holders. Safety and Health Information Bulletin (SHIB), October 15, 2003.

Occupational Safety and Health Administration (OSHA): Disposal of Contaminated Needles and Blood Tube Holders Used in Phlebotomy. Safety and Health Information Bulletin (SHIB), October 15, 2003, http://www.osha.gov/dts/shib/shib101503.html.

Procedures for examination and certification: Patient's bill of rights. (1973). *Hospitals, 47,* (February), 41.

Rizzo, D. C. (2001). Delmar's *Fundamentals of anatomy and physiology*. Clifton Park, NY: Delmar, Cengage Learning.

Seeley, R. R., Stephens, T. D., & Tate, P. (1991). *Essentials of anatomy and physiology.* St. Louis: Mosby Year Book.

Seigworth, G. R. (1980). Bloodletting over the centuries. *New York State Journal of Medicine,* (December), 2022–2027.

Webster's new international dictionary of the English language. (1989). New York: Windsor Court.

Wilmot, J., & Wilmot, W. (1985). *Interpersonal conflict.* Dubuque, IA: Wm. C. Brown.

Glossary

A

access—availability

accommodator—one who aids, assists

aerobic—living in the presence of air/oxygen

airborne precautions—use of protective devices that reduce the spread of airborne droplet transmission of infectious agents

amylase—an enzyme that converts starch into sugar

anaerobic—living without air/oxygen

antecubital—before the crease of the forearm and upper arm

anticoagulant—any agent that prevents coagulation

antigen—a substance that creates an antibody when introduced into blood or tissue

aorta—the largest artery that carries blood from the heart to be distributed by branch arteries through the body

arterial puncture—puncture of the radial, femoral, or brachial artery with the purpose of obtaining an arterial blood sample for testing pH, O_2, and CO_2

arteriole—the small terminal branch of an artery that ends in capillaries

arteriotomy—an incision into an artery

artery—a tubular, muscular, and elastic-walled vessel that carries blood from the heart through the body

articulation—speaking in a distinct, clear manner

ASAP—as soon as possible

aseptic—free from infection

atherosclerosis—a disease in which arteries are severely narrowed by lipid deposits on the inner walls

atria—the two chambers of the heart that receive blood from the veins and force it into the ventricles

autoimmune—rising from and against the body's own tissues

avoider—one who shuns, bypasses, evades

B

bacteremia—the presence of bacteria in the circulating blood

basilic vein—prominent vein of the forearm located on the inside edge of the antecubital fossa.

battery—intentionally touching a person without authorization to do so

Betadine—an iodine solution

bevel—the slanted edge at the tip of a needle

bile—a yellow or greenish liquid secreted by the liver that aids in digestion

bilirubin—a reddish-yellow pigment in urine, blood, or bile

bloodborne pathogens—pathogenic microorganisms that can be present in blood and can cause disease

butterfly needle—a needle and tubing connected with a plastic wing-shaped holder that is used for fragile veins; it may be used attached to a syringe or with a luer adapter

C

CAP (College of American Pathologists)—a medical society comprised exclusively of pathologists serving over 15,000 physician members and the laboratory community worldwide that is widely considered the leader in providing laboratory quality improvement programs

capillary—a small blood vessel connecting arterioles with venules

capillary action—the process by which blood automatically flows into a thin tube during a capillary blood collection procedure

capillary puncture—also called a skin puncture; this refers to puncturing the skin by means of a lancet to obtain a blood sample. This sample is a mixture of blood from arterioles, venules, and capillaries.

CDC (Centers for Disease Control and Prevention)—an agency of the Department of Health and Human Services. Its function is to promote health and quality of life by preventing and controlling disease, injury, and disability

central venous catheter—an artificial line placed into the patient's body with the purpose of obtaining blood samples, administering drugs, supplying nutrition, and transfusing blood products

cephalic vein—prominent vein in the forearm utilized for venipuncture

circulatory system—the system that comprises blood, blood vessels, lymphatics, and heart, and is concerned with the circulation of the blood and lymph

cirrhosis—inflammation of an organ, particularly the liver

CLIA 1988—the Clinical Laboratory Improvement Amendments of 1988, mandating that all laboratories must be regulated according to the same standards, regardless of location, type, or size

clot—a clump of material formed out of the contents of blood

CLSI (Clinical and Laboratory Standards Institute; formerly NCCLS)—an institute that sets standards for specimen collection and handling to protect the patient from injury and negative outcomes

coagulation—cessation of bleeding; formation of a clot. The clotting process consists of the action of blood vessels, platelets, and coagulation factors

colitis—inflammation of the colon

collaborator—one who assists, acts as a partner

communication—the transmission of information

competence—proficiency, skill, knowledge

compromiser—one who adapts, adjusts, negotiates

confidentiality—the protected right of health professionals not to disclose information pertaining to a client that is obtained during the delivery of health care services

conflict—clash, confrontation, difference, opposition, unrest

contact precautions—protective measures that reduce the risk of transmission of diseases through direct or indirect contact

contaminated—referring to the presence of blood or infectious material on an item or surface

controller—one who rules, manages

courtesy—respect, consideration, attention, manners, politeness

credibility—integrity, trustworthiness, honesty

cupping—a technique of bloodletting in which a vacuum is induced into a cup or glass. The glass is placed over the skin and the vacuum brings blood to the surface. The skin is cut and blood is allowed to flow.

customer—anyone to whom a service or a product is provided

cyanotic—displaying blueness of the skin, as from imperfectly oxygenated blood

cytopathology—the science involved with disease at the cellular level

D

decontamination—the use of physical or chemical means to destroy bloodborne pathogens on a surface to the point where they are no longer able to transmit infectious particles

deontology—an ethical theory based on moral obligation or commitment to others

diastole—the resting phase of the heart muscle's contraction

distal—situated away from the center of the body

dorsal—relating to the back side

droplet precautions—protective measures that produce the risk of transmission of diseases that can be transmitted through contact with mucous membrane of the nose, mouth, or eyes

E

edematous—swollen due to an accumulation of excess fluid in the tissue

egoism—an ethical theory that considers self-interest the goal of all human actions

embolus—an abnormal particle (like an air bubble) circulating in the blood

engineering controls—physical and mechanical devices designed to reduce or eliminate the hazards of transferring potentially infectious diseases

enzymes—protein substances produced by living cells; they are essential to life, as they act as catalysts in metabolism

erythrocyte—red blood cell

ethics—an area of philosophy that examines values, actions, and choices to determine right and wrong etiology—the science and study of diseases and their causes and origins

evacuated collection system—a venous blood collection system that involves a double-pointed needle and vacuumized collection tubes. The vacuum draws blood into the tube

excretory organs—organs that discharge wastes from the body

external customer—someone to whom a service is provided who is not employed by the health care facility

F

filtrates—fluid that remains after a liquid is passed through a membranous filter

G

gauge—needle bore size

gauze—loosely woven cotton fabric, available in sterile packets

granulocyte—a cell with granule-containing cytoplasm

H

HBV—hepatitis B virus

HCV—hepatitis C virus

hematoma—a swelling or mass of blood, usually clotted, in an organ or tissue, caused by a ruptured blood vessel due to injury

hematopoiesis—the formation of blood cells in the body

hemochromatosis—a disorder of iron metabolism

hemoconcentration—increased localized blood concentration of molecules such as cells, proteins, and coagulation factors

hemoglobin—an iron-containing protein pigment present in red blood cells. It functions primarily to transport oxygen from the lungs to the tissues of the body

hemostasis—the process of coagulation, or clot formation, that repairs vessel damage and stops blood loss

heparin—a drug used as an anticoagulant

HICPAC (Healthcare Infection Control Practices Advisory Committee)—a committee whose primary function is to issue recommendations for preventing and controlling nosocomial infections in the form of guidelines, resolutions, and informal communications

HIPPA (Health Insurance Portability and Accountability Act)—a federal protection law for the privacy of health insurance

histopathology—science involved with the disease of tissue

HIV—human immunodeficiency virus

hub—clear, plastic section of the needle

humors—fluids in the body

I

insulin—hormone that regulates the metabolism of glucose

internal customer—someone to whom a service is provided who is an employee of the health care facility

interstitial fluid—fluid between the tissues

J

JCAHO (Joint Commission on Accreditation of Healthcare Organizations)— Now known as the Joint Commission. An independent, not-for-profit organization that evaluates and accredits health care organizations in the United States

L

lancet—a small surgical blade used to puncture the skin

lateral—referring to the side

latex allergy—an allergic reaction that can result from repeated exposures to proteins in natural rubber latex through skin contact or inhalation

leech—a blood-sucking worm utilized in bloodletting

leukocyte—white blood cell

ligate—to tie a blood vessel with silk thread, wire, or filament to stop bleeding

listening—paying attention, making an effort to hear and understand

loyalty—firm allegiance

lymphocyte—a leukocyte produced in the lymphoid tissue; lymphocytes are the cellular elements of lymph and play a role in the body's immune system

lymphostasis—lack of fluid drainage in the lymph system; stoppage of lymph flow

M

median cubital vein—vein in the antecubital area that is most commonly used for venipuncture

message—any communication, written or oral, from one person to another

monocyte—a large leukocyte formed in bone marrow, with abundant cytoplasm and a kidney-shaped nucleus; ingests bacteria and debris in tissues

morning rounds—a batch of laboratory test orders scheduled for early morning collection

N

Needlestick Safety and Prevention Act—a bill signed November 6, 2000, that contains an amendment to OSHA's bloodborne pathogen standard to ensure more widespread use of safer medical devices to prevent dangerous needlesticks. The legislation requires employers to identify and provide safer equipment for their staffs

nephron—structural and functional unit of the kidney

neutrophil—leukocyte that engulfs and digests pathogens found in tissues. Its granules stain with neither basic nor acid dyes

NIOSH (National Institute for Occupational Safety and Health)—a federal agency responsible for conducting research and making recommendations for the prevention of work-related disease and injury. It is part of the Centers for Disease Control and Prevention

nosocomial—a disorder associated with being treated in a hospital, but unrelated to the patient's primary condition

O

obligationism—an ethical theory that attempts to resolve ethical dilemmas by balancing distributive justice with the promotion of good and the prevention of harm

occult—hidden

OSHA (Occupational Safety and Health Administration)—a federal agency that develops and promotes occupational safety and health standards, develops and issues regulations, conducts investigations and inspections, and issues citations and proposes penalties for noncompliance with safety and health standards and regulations

osteomyelitis—an inflammatory disease of the bone, resulting from infection

P

pathogens—disease-producing agents

patient-focused care—an approach to health care in which services are simplified, decentralized, and placed close to the patient

Patient's Bill of Rights—a protection of rights for the health care patient, such as the rights to human dignity, privacy, confidentiality, informed consent, and refusal of treatment

peripheral circulation—includes both the systemic circulation and the pulmonary circulation

personal protective equipment (PPE)— specialized clothing or equipment worn by a professional for protection against a hazard.

phenylalanine—amino acid essential for the growth in children and for the metabolism of protein

phlebotomist—an individual trained and skilled in obtaining blood samples for clinical testing

plantar—relating to the sole of the foot

plasma—the yellow fluid component of blood

point-of-care testing—collection of a blood sample and immediate testing at the site of client care

polycythemia—abnormal increase in the number of erythrocytes in the blood

portal vein—a short vein that receives branches from several veins leading from abdominal organs and then enters the liver

pulmonary circulation— the flow of blood to the lungs

Q

quality assurance—established policies and procedures to ensure that laboratory testing is carefully monitored from beginning to end, including collection of specimens

R

reflective listening—repeating what has been heard back to the speaker

reliability—accurate, dependable performance

respiratory system—consists of the nose, nasal cavity, pharynx, larynx, trachea, bronchi, and lungs

responsiveness—readiness to provide prompt service

risk management—the monitoring of patterns and trends in the health care environment to assure the safety of patients and professionals

routine collection—orders collected per individual laboratory policy

S

saline—a solution containing sodium chloride used as a plasma substitute and a means to correct electrolyte imbalances

security—assurance, certainty, safety

septicemia—the presence in the bloodstream of infectious microorganisms or their toxins

sharp—an object that can penetrate the skin such as a needle, scalpel, broken glass, broken capillary tube, or lancet

social contract theory—an ethical theory based on the assumption that the least advantaged are the norm, with income, liberty, opportunity, and self-respect distributed equally

standard precautions—combines many of the basic principles of universal precautions with techniques of body substance isolation

stat—at once, immediately. From the Latin word *statim*

sterilize—to use a physical or chemical procedure to destroy all microbial life

syringe—a device used for drawing out (or injecting) a quantity of fluid

systemic circulation—the flow of blood to the body, exclusive of the pulmonary circulation

systole—the active, or contracting, phase of the heart muscle's contraction; the upper number of a blood pressure reading

T

tangibles—things that are actual and concrete

teamwork—the subordination of the individual's tasks or goals to the common purpose of the group

teleology—an ethical theory that determines right or good based on an action's consequences

tetany—a disorder characterized by muscular twitching, cramps, and convulsions

thrombocyte—platelet

thromboplastin—a lipoprotein that promotes blood clotting; found in platelets

thrombosed—occluded, or blocked, by a blood clot

thrombus—a clot of blood formed within a blood vessel and remaining attached to its point of origin

timed collection—orders collected at a specified collection time

tourniquet—a length of rubber or synthetic rubber tied around the arm to arrest blood flow and increase venous filling

tunica adventitia—an enclosing tissue that makes up the outer layer of the artery wall

tunica intima—the innermost membrane of the artery wall

tunica media—the middle layer of the artery wall

U

understanding—appreciation, sensitivity, comprehension

universal body substance precautions—an approach to infection control that considers all human blood and certain body fluids to be infectious and handles them as such infectious

urinary system—consists of the kidneys, ureters, urinary bladder, and urethra

urine—fluid secreted by the kidneys

urobilinogen—compound formed in the intestine from the breakdown of bilirubin

V

values—strongly held personal and professional beliefs about worth and importance

vein—a vessel that carries blood back to the heart

venipuncture—a puncture of a vein with the purpose of withdrawing blood

ventricles—the two chambers of the heart that receive blood from the corresponding atria and force it into the arteries

venule—a small vein connecting the capillaries with the larger systemic veins

Index